CHAIR PILATES FOR BEGINNERS

Mary Dixon

TABLE OF CONTENT

CHAPTER ONE 5

Introduction to Chair Pilates 5

Understanding Chair Pilates 10

Benefits of Chair Pilates 16

Preparing Your Workspace............................... 19

Safety Considerations 22

CHAPTER TWO 27

Essential Chair Pilates Exercises 27

Seated Posture and Alignment.......................... 31

Breathing Techniques 36

Warm-up Exercises.. 41

Core Strengthening Exercises 44

Upper Body Exercises...................................... 48

Lower Body Exercises 51

Cool-down Stretches.. 55

CHAPTER THREE 59

Chair Pilates Routines for Beginners................. 59

Morning Chair Pilates Routine 64

Midday Energy Booster 67

Evening Relaxation Sequence 70

Chair Pilates for Posture Improvement 73

Chair Pilates for Stress Relief 77

CHAPTER FOUR 81

Chair Pilates for Wellness 81

Chair Pilates and Stress Reduction 86

Chair Pilates for Back Pain Relief 89

Chair Pilates for Improved Posture 94

Chair Pilates for Increased Flexibility 99

CHAPTER FIVE 109

Chair Pilates Progression and Advanced Techniques . 109

Building Strength and Flexibility 113

Advanced Chair Pilates Exercises 118

Chair Pilates for Specific Goals 122

Maintaining a Regular Practice 127

CONCLUSION 135

CHAPTER ONE

Introduction to Chair Pilates

In today's fast-paced world, where our lives often revolve around hectic schedules and demanding responsibilities, finding a way to maintain our physical and mental well-being is paramount. Chair Pilates, a gentle yet highly effective form of exercise, emerges as an accessible and versatile solution for individuals seeking a holistic approach to health and fitness.

Combining elements of traditional Pilates with the convenience of a chair, this practice provides a pathway to improved strength, flexibility, posture, and overall vitality. In this introductory exploration of Chair Pilates, we will delve into the origins, principles, benefits, and unique characteristics of this practice, shedding light on why it has become a popular choice for individuals of all ages and fitness levels.

Origins and Evolution of Chair Pilates

Pilates, as a discipline, was developed by Joseph Pilates during the early 20th century. Originally named "Contrology," Pilates focused on the art of controlled movements and the utilization of the mind to guide the body. Joseph Pilates' holistic approach was rooted in the belief that physical and mental health are interdependent. While his method involved exercises on the mat, he also designed a series of apparatuses to facilitate and intensify the movements. One such apparatus was the "Wunda Chair," which has now become synonymous with Chair Pilates.

Over time, Chair Pilates has evolved and adapted to meet the needs of a broader audience. It has gained popularity among individuals with varying levels of fitness and physical abilities. The chair provides support, stability, and adaptability, making it an ideal choice for both beginners and experienced practitioners. This adaptability allows individuals to perform a wide range of exercises while sitting or standing, making it an inclusive fitness practice.

The Principles of Chair Pilates

At the core of Chair Pilates are six fundamental principles: concentration, control, centering, precision, breath, and flow. These principles guide every movement and exercise, facilitating the development of physical awareness and mindfulness.

1. Concentration: Chair Pilates requires focused attention on each movement, fostering a strong mind-body connection. By being fully present in the moment, individuals can maximize the benefits of each exercise.

2. Control: Controlled and deliberate movements are essential in Chair Pilates. Practitioners learn to utilize specific muscle groups while avoiding unnecessary tension in others, allowing for improved muscular control.

3. Centering: At the center of Chair Pilates lies the concept of the body's "powerhouse," encompassing the abdominal muscles, lower back, pelvic floor, and hips. Strengthening this core area is key to maintaining stability and balance in daily life.

4. Precision: Precision is the hallmark of Pilates. Exercises are designed to be precise, efficient, and tailored to the individual's needs, which helps in preventing injury and promoting optimal results.

5. Breath: Proper breathing is vital in Chair Pilates. The practice emphasizes coordinated breathing techniques that facilitate the flow of oxygen to the muscles, enhancing endurance and promoting relaxation.

6. Flow: A continuous flow of movement is a key aspect of Chair Pilates. This emphasis on fluidity ensures that exercises are executed with grace and rhythm, promoting balance, flexibility, and strength.

Benefits of Chair Pilates

Chair Pilates offers a myriad of benefits that extend beyond physical fitness. Its low-impact nature makes it suitable for individuals of all ages and fitness levels. Here are some of the advantages of incorporating Chair Pilates into your life:

1. Improved Posture: Chair Pilates strengthens the core muscles that support the spine, promoting better alignment and posture. This can alleviate back pain and reduce the risk of injury.

2. Enhanced Flexibility: The practice includes stretching and flexibility exercises that can increase range of motion and reduce muscle tightness.

3. Increased Strength: Chair Pilates focuses on building both core and peripheral muscle strength, providing a full-body workout.

4. Stress Reduction: The mind-body connection inherent in Chair Pilates promotes relaxation and reduces stress. Focused breathing and mindfulness techniques contribute to improved mental well-being.

5. Better Balance: The chair provides stability, making it an excellent choice for individuals working on balance and coordination.

6. Accessible for All: Chair Pilates can be adapted to suit various physical abilities and limitations, making it accessible to a broad range of individuals.

In this introduction to Chair Pilates, we have touched upon its origins, principles, and numerous benefits. Chair Pilates is not merely a form of exercise but a holistic approach to wellness that promotes physical and mental health.

Whether you are a seasoned fitness enthusiast or a beginner seeking a path to greater well-being, Chair Pilates offers a versatile and adaptable journey towards improved strength, flexibility, and vitality. In the chapters that follow, we will delve deeper into the specifics of Chair Pilates, providing a comprehensive guide for beginners and experienced practitioners alike.

Understanding Chair Pilates

Chair Pilates is a dynamic and adaptable exercise system that combines the principles of traditional Pilates with the added dimension of a specialized chair apparatus.

This unique form of fitness provides a comprehensive workout that focuses on strengthening the body's core, enhancing flexibility, improving posture, and cultivating overall well-being. In this exploration, we will delve deeper into the understanding of Chair Pilates, its components, benefits, and how it has become an increasingly popular choice for individuals seeking a balanced and holistic approach to physical fitness.

The Chair Pilates Apparatus

At the heart of Chair Pilates lies the chair apparatus itself. This specialized piece of equipment, often referred to as the "Wunda Chair," was originally designed by Joseph Pilates as part of his pioneering exercise system. Today, modern adaptations of the chair have made it more accessible and user-friendly. The chair features a padded seat, a set of springs, handles, and a frame that allows for a wide range of exercises to be performed.

The chair's primary function is to provide resistance, support, and stability as individuals engage in various movements and exercises.

Its versatility enables practitioners to perform both seated and standing exercises, accommodating a wide spectrum of physical abilities and fitness levels.

The chair apparatus, in combination with the principles of Pilates, fosters an environment of controlled, precise, and low-impact movements that target specific muscle groups.

Key Principles of Chair Pilates

Chair Pilates adheres to the foundational principles of traditional Pilates, which include concentration, control, centering, precision, breath, and flow.

These principles guide the practice and provide a framework for mindful and effective exercise.

1. Concentration: Chair Pilates emphasizes the importance of concentration.

Practitioners must remain fully engaged in each exercise, ensuring that movements are executed with intention and awareness.

2. Control: Control is a central element in Chair Pilates. Movements are performed with precision, ensuring that muscles are engaged and released in a controlled manner, reducing the risk of injury.

3. Centering: At the core of Chair Pilates is the concept of the body's powerhouse, which includes the abdominal muscles, lower back, pelvic floor, and hips. Strengthening this area is essential for maintaining stability and balance.

4. Precision: Precision is a hallmark of Chair Pilates. Exercises are designed to be exact, efficient, and tailored to individual needs. This approach prevents unnecessary strain and promotes optimal results.

5. Breath: Proper breathing is vital in Chair Pilates. The practice places a strong emphasis on coordinated breathing techniques that enhance the flow of oxygen to the muscles, improving endurance and relaxation.

6. Flow: A continuous flow of movement is a key aspect of Chair Pilates. Exercises are executed with grace and rhythm, ensuring that they are connected and harmonious.

The Benefits of Chair Pilates

Chair Pilates offers a wide array of benefits that encompass physical, mental, and emotional well-being. Some of the notable advantages include:

1. **Enhanced Core Strength:** Chair Pilates places significant emphasis on strengthening the core muscles, which are vital for overall stability and posture.

2. **Improved Flexibility:** Through a combination of stretching and flexibility exercises, Chair Pilates can increase the range of motion, alleviating muscle stiffness.

3. **Better Posture:** The practice encourages proper alignment, leading to improved posture and reduced risk of back pain.

4. **Stress Reduction:** Chair Pilates incorporates mindfulness and controlled breathing techniques that promote relaxation and stress relief.

5. **Balanced Muscle Development:** Exercises in Chair Pilates target both the core and peripheral muscles, providing a balanced and well-rounded workout.

6. Enhanced Balance and Coordination: The chair apparatus offers support and stability, making it an ideal choice for those looking to improve balance and coordination.

7. Accessible for All Ages: Chair Pilates can be adapted to suit various physical abilities and age groups, making it accessible to a wide range of individuals.

Who Can Benefit from Chair Pilates?

One of the key strengths of Chair Pilates is its accessibility. This practice is suitable for individuals of all ages, fitness levels, and physical abilities. Whether you are a senior looking to maintain mobility and balance, an office worker seeking relief from the strains of sedentary work, or an athlete aiming to improve core strength and flexibility, Chair Pilates can be tailored to meet your specific needs.

For those with physical limitations or recovering from injuries, Chair Pilates provides a gentle yet effective means of rehabilitation and recovery. The chair apparatus allows for modifications, making it possible to work around physical restrictions while building strength and flexibility.

Moreover, Chair Pilates serves as an excellent complement to other forms of exercise and wellness practices. Whether you are a dedicated yogi, a runner, or a weightlifter, incorporating Chair Pilates into your routine can enhance your overall performance and reduce the risk of injury.

Chair Pilates is a versatile and all-encompassing fitness practice that offers numerous advantages for individuals seeking a balanced approach to physical well-being.

By combining the principles of traditional Pilates with the chair apparatus, this form of exercise promotes strength, flexibility, posture, and relaxation. Its accessibility and adaptability make it an excellent choice for individuals of all ages and fitness levels.

Whether you are a beginner embarking on your fitness journey or an experienced practitioner looking to enhance your core strength and flexibility, Chair Pilates offers a path to holistic well-being. In the chapters that follow, we will delve deeper into the essential components, exercises, and routines of Chair Pilates, providing you with a comprehensive guide to this beneficial and transformative practice.

Benefits of Chair Pilates

Chair Pilates is a highly beneficial form of exercise that offers a wide range of advantages for individuals of all ages and fitness levels. This practice combines the principles of traditional Pilates with a specialized chair apparatus, providing support, stability, and versatility. Here are some of the key benefits of Chair Pilates:

1. Improved Core Strength: Chair Pilates places a strong emphasis on strengthening the core muscles, including the abdominals, lower back, pelvic floor, and hips. This results in enhanced stability and better posture, reducing the risk of back pain and injury.

2. Enhanced Flexibility: Through a combination of stretching and flexibility exercises, Chair Pilates increases the range of motion in the joints and muscles. This can alleviate muscle tightness and improve overall flexibility.

3. Better Posture: Chair Pilates promotes proper alignment and awareness of body positioning. By strengthening the muscles that support the spine, it helps individuals maintain better posture, reducing the risk of slouching and its associated problems.

4. Stress Reduction: Chair Pilates incorporates mindfulness and controlled breathing techniques that promote relaxation and reduce stress. The focus on mind-body connection can lead to a calmer and more centered state of mind.

5. Balanced Muscle Development: Chair Pilates targets both the core muscles and peripheral muscle groups. This balanced approach ensures that all areas of the body are developed harmoniously, reducing the risk of muscle imbalances.

6. Enhanced Balance and Coordination: The chair apparatus provides support and stability, making it an ideal choice for individuals looking to improve balance and coordination. This is especially beneficial for seniors and those at risk of falls.

7. Low-Impact Exercise: Chair Pilates is gentle on the joints and is considered a low-impact form of exercise. This makes it suitable for individuals with joint pain, arthritis, or those recovering from injuries.

8. Accessible for All Ages: One of the notable strengths of Chair Pilates is its accessibility.

It can be adapted to suit various physical abilities and age groups, making it suitable for individuals of all ages, from children to seniors.

9. Rehabilitation and Injury Prevention: For those with physical limitations or recovering from injuries, Chair Pilates provides a gentle yet effective means of rehabilitation and recovery. The chair apparatus allows for modifications, making it possible to work around physical restrictions while building strength and flexibility.

10. Complement to Other Exercise Practices: Chair Pilates serves as an excellent complement to other forms of exercise and wellness practices. Whether you are a dedicated yogi, a runner, or a weightlifter, incorporating Chair Pilates into your routine can enhance your overall performance, reduce the risk of injury, and provide a balanced approach to fitness.

11. Mind-Body Connection: The focus on concentration, control, and mindfulness in Chair Pilates encourages individuals to become more attuned to their bodies. This can lead to a heightened awareness of how the body moves and feels, promoting overall well-being.

12. Improved Breathing: Chair Pilates places a strong emphasis on proper breathing techniques. Practitioners learn to coordinate their breath with movement, promoting optimal oxygen intake and increased endurance.

In conclusion, Chair Pilates is a versatile and adaptable exercise practice that offers a multitude of benefits for individuals seeking to improve their physical and mental well-being. Its accessibility, low-impact nature, and focus on core strength, flexibility, posture, and stress reduction make it a valuable addition to a holistic wellness routine.

Whether you are looking to build core strength, alleviate back pain, or simply maintain a healthier, more balanced lifestyle, Chair Pilates has something to offer individuals of all backgrounds and fitness levels.

Preparing Your Workspace

Preparing your workspace is an essential aspect of practicing Chair Pilates safely and effectively. Creating a comfortable and organized environment can contribute to your overall well-being during your exercise routine. Here are some key considerations when preparing your workspace for Chair Pilates:

1. Select a Quiet and Well-Lit Area: Choose a quiet and well-lit space for your Chair Pilates practice. Natural light can be particularly beneficial, as it creates a positive and energizing atmosphere.

2. Clear the Area: Remove any obstacles or clutter from the floor surrounding your chair to prevent accidents or tripping during your exercises.

3. Place Your Chair: Position your Chair Pilates apparatus in a location where it has sufficient space around it. Ensure that the chair is stable and on a flat surface.

4. Check the Chair: Before each practice session, inspect your chair for any signs of wear or damage, such as loose screws or instability. A stable chair is essential for your safety during exercises.

5. Use a Mat or Towel: Placing a yoga or exercise mat beneath your chair can provide cushioning and prevent the chair from slipping on the floor. Alternatively, you can use a folded towel to protect your feet and reduce the impact on your joints.

6. Comfortable Clothing: Wear comfortable and breathable clothing that allows for ease of movement.

Tight or restrictive clothing can hinder your ability to perform Chair Pilates exercises.

7. Water and Towel: Have a bottle of water nearby to stay hydrated during your practice. Keep a small towel handy for wiping away sweat if needed.

8. Supportive Footwear: Many Chair Pilates exercises are performed barefoot, but if you prefer to wear footwear, choose shoes with non-slip soles that provide stability.

9. Consider Music: Some individuals find that soft, calming music enhances their Chair Pilates experience by creating a relaxed and focused ambiance. Consider playing your favorite soothing tunes in the background.

10. Limit Distractions: Turn off or silence your phone and eliminate other potential distractions to create a peaceful and undisturbed space for your practice.

11. Personalize Your Space: Add personal touches to your workout area. This could include inspirational quotes, plants, or any other items that create a sense of comfort and motivation. By paying attention to these workspace preparations, you can ensure a safe, comfortable, and enjoyable Chair Pilates experience.

A well-organized and inviting space can enhance your focus and commitment to your practice, making it easier to reap the many benefits of Chair Pilates.

Safety Considerations

Ensuring safety during your Chair Pilates practice is of paramount importance. While Chair Pilates is a low-impact exercise that is generally safe for most individuals, it's crucial to take certain precautions to prevent injuries and maintain your well-being. Here are some safety considerations to keep in mind when practicing Chair Pilates:

1. Consult Your Healthcare Provider: Before beginning any exercise program, including Chair Pilates, it's advisable to consult with your healthcare provider, especially if you have any pre-existing medical conditions or concerns. They can offer guidance and ensure that Chair Pilates is a suitable choice for your individual health and fitness needs.

2. Proper Warm-Up: Always start your Chair Pilates session with a gentle warm-up. Warm-up exercises help prepare your muscles and joints for more intense movements, reducing the risk of strains or injuries.

3. Follow Proper Form: Pay close attention to your posture and body alignment during each exercise. Following the principles of Chair Pilates, such as centering and control, is essential. Proper form ensures that you target the intended muscle groups and minimizes the risk of injury.

4. Listen to Your Body: Tune in to your body's signals. If an exercise causes pain, discomfort, or strain, stop immediately and assess your form. It's essential to distinguish between muscle engagement and pain due to improper technique.

5. Start Slowly: If you're new to Chair Pilates or returning after a break, start with the basics and easier exercises. Gradually increase the intensity and complexity of your routine as your strength and skill improve.

6. Use Props Mindfully: Some Chair Pilates exercises involve additional props or resistance bands. Use these props carefully and make sure they are secure to avoid accidents or injuries.

7. Controlled Movements: Avoid rapid, jerky movements. Chair Pilates focuses on controlled, precise motions. Quick or erratic movements can increase the risk of strain or injury.

8. Be Mindful of Overexertion: Avoid overexertion or pushing yourself too hard. Pay attention to your body's limits and respect your current fitness level. Progress should be gradual to prevent overuse injuries.

9. Breath Awareness: Incorporate proper breathing techniques into your practice. Breathing in sync with your movements helps with oxygen intake and reduces the risk of dizziness or discomfort.

10. Stay Hydrated: Keep a bottle of water nearby and stay hydrated during your practice. Dehydration can affect your performance and well-being.

11. Avoid Holding Your Breath: Holding your breath during exercises can increase tension and reduce the effectiveness of your practice. Focus on maintaining steady and controlled breathing.

12. Watch for Dizziness or Lightheadedness: If you start to feel dizzy or lightheaded during your Chair Pilates session, stop immediately, sit down, and take deep breaths. These sensations may indicate a drop in blood pressure.

13. Personalize Your Practice Modify exercises to suit your individual needs and limitations.

If you have specific health concerns or physical restrictions, work with a qualified instructor who can help tailor your Chair Pilates routine accordingly.

14. Cool Down and Stretch: Finish your Chair Pilates practice with a cool-down period that includes gentle stretches. This helps to release tension and prevents post-workout muscle soreness.

15. Seek Professional Guidance: If you're new to Chair Pilates or have specific health concerns, consider working with a certified Chair Pilates instructor who can provide guidance, correct your form, and ensure that your practice is safe and effective.

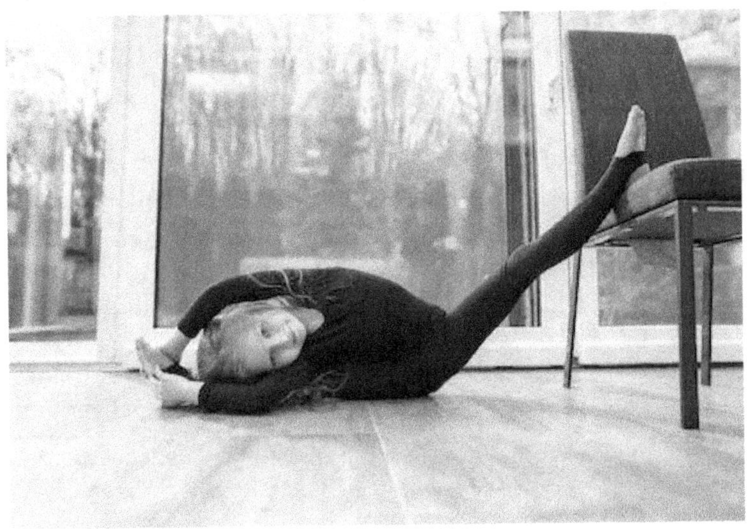

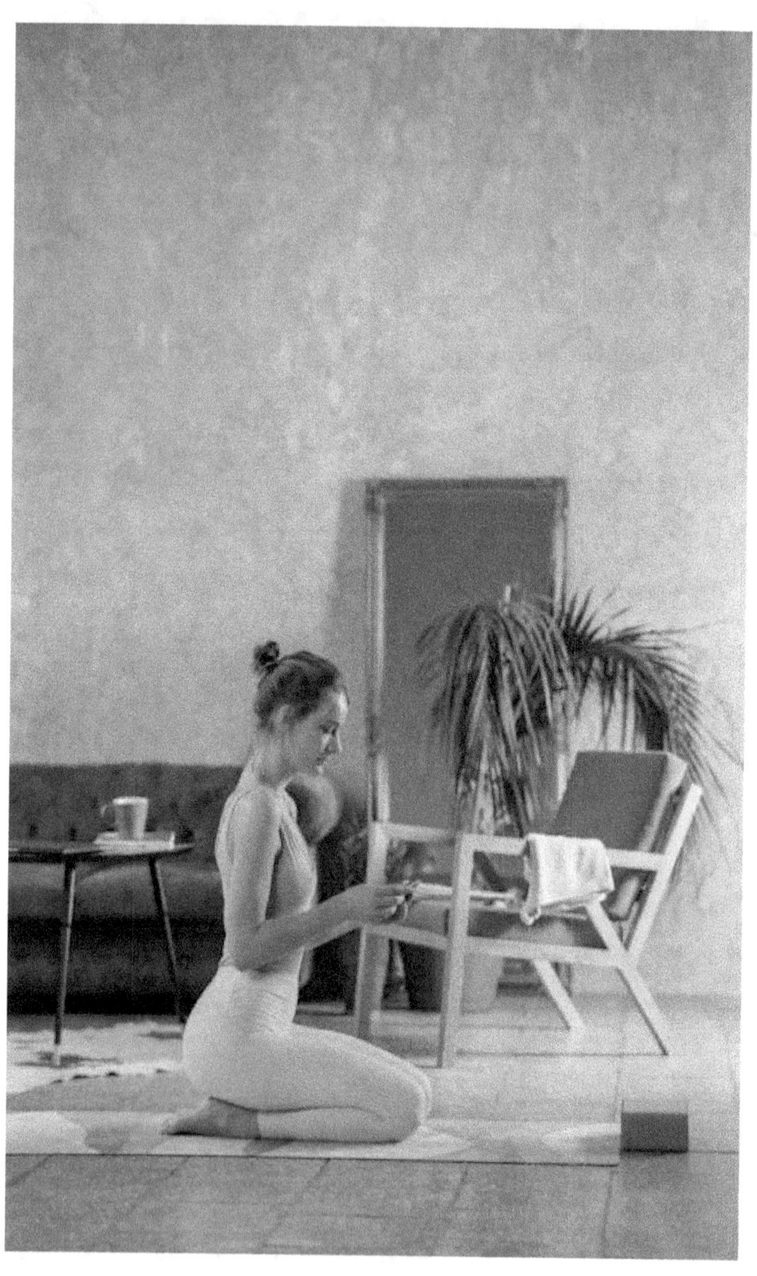

CHAPTER TWO

Essential Chair Pilates Exercises

In the quest for a well-rounded fitness routine that promotes core strength, flexibility, balance, and overall well-being, Chair Pilates emerges as a highly effective and adaptable practice.

By combining the principles of traditional Pilates with the convenience of a specialized chair apparatus, Chair Pilates offers a comprehensive workout that can be tailored to individuals of all ages and fitness levels.

This introductory exploration delves into the world of Chair Pilates, specifically focusing on essential exercises that form the foundation of this versatile and rewarding fitness practice.

The Power of Chair Pilates

Chair Pilates, often associated with the "Wunda Chair," is a dynamic approach to exercise that has its roots in the pioneering work of Joseph Pilates during the early 20th century. Joseph Pilates originally designed the chair apparatus as part of his comprehensive exercise system, known as "Contrology," which aimed to create a balanced development of the body and mind.

Chair Pilates is distinguished by its focus on controlled, precise, and low-impact movements. These exercises are designed to engage specific muscle groups while maintaining proper posture and alignment.

The chair apparatus provides support, resistance, and stability, making it an ideal choice for individuals looking to strengthen their core, enhance flexibility, and improve their overall physical and mental well-being.

The essential exercises in Chair Pilates serve as building blocks for a strong and balanced body. They are integral to the practice's core principles, which include concentration, control, centering, precision, breath, and flow.

These principles guide each movement, fostering a heightened awareness of the mind-body connection and promoting a safe and effective workout.

The Essential Exercises

Here, we will explore some of the fundamental Chair Pilates exercises that lay the groundwork for a holistic fitness routine. These exercises encompass a range of movements that target various muscle groups, offering a balanced workout for the entire body. Whether you're a beginner or an experienced practitioner, these essential exercises can be customized to your skill level and fitness goals.

1. Chair Squats: Chair squats are a fantastic way to strengthen the lower body. They engage the quadriceps, hamstrings, and glutes while promoting balance and stability. This exercise helps in improving leg strength and overall mobility.

2. Seated Leg Lifts: Seated leg lifts focus on the quadriceps and abdominal muscles. They encourage controlled movements and enhance core strength. These exercises also promote proper posture and alignment.

3. Arm Circles: Arm circles help in increasing shoulder flexibility and improving posture. They engage the deltoids and upper back muscles, promoting upper body strength and flexibility.

4. Spine Stretch: The spine stretch exercise is ideal for enhancing flexibility in the back and hamstrings.

It encourages spinal mobility and helps in achieving better posture.

5. Single-Leg Stretch: Single-leg stretch is a core-focused exercise that targets the abdominals. It promotes control and balance while strengthening the core muscles.

6. Swan Dive: The swan dive exercise is excellent for strengthening the back, shoulders, and glutes. It encourages spinal extension and flexibility.

7. Mermaid Stretch: Mermaid stretches help improve lateral flexibility and balance. They engage the oblique muscles and offer a sense of elongation and freedom in the body.

8. Pelvic Lift: Pelvic lifts are core-strengthening exercises that target the abdominals and lower back. They encourage proper alignment and balance.

9. Footwork Footwork exercises enhance leg strength and flexibility. They engage the calf and thigh muscles while improving ankle mobility.

10. Breathing Exercises: Breathing exercises are an integral part of Chair Pilates, promoting mindful breathing and oxygenation of the body. They assist in relaxation and concentration during the practice.

These essential Chair Pilates exercises are foundational to the practice, providing a comprehensive full-body workout that focuses on core strength, flexibility, and improved posture. Whether you are new to Chair Pilates or a seasoned practitioner, these exercises can be tailored to your needs and fitness level, offering a pathway to a healthier, more balanced, and agile body.

Seated Posture and Alignment

Seated Posture and Alignment in Chair Pilates

Seated posture and alignment are fundamental aspects of Chair Pilates, providing the foundation for a safe and effective practice. In Chair Pilates, the chair apparatus serves as both a support and a challenge, encouraging individuals to engage their core muscles, maintain proper alignment, and achieve a sense of balance and stability.

Understanding and mastering seated posture and alignment is key to reaping the full benefits of Chair Pilates. This exploration will guide you through the principles and techniques for achieving optimal seated posture and alignment.

The Importance of Seated Posture and Alignment

In Chair Pilates, seated posture and alignment serve several critical purposes:

1. Core Engagement: Maintaining proper seated posture engages the core muscles, including the abdominals and lower back. This not only strengthens the core but also promotes overall stability.

2. Spinal Health: Good seated posture supports the natural curvature of the spine, reducing the risk of strain or injury to the back. It encourages a healthy spine and minimizes the potential for discomfort.

3. Efficiency of Movement: Correct alignment ensures that you target the intended muscle groups during exercises, leading to a more efficient and effective workout.

4. Mind-Body Connection: Seated posture and alignment are intimately connected to the principles of concentration and control in Chair Pilates.

Being aware of your body's positioning fosters a strong mind-body connection and mindfulness during your practice.

Achieving Optimal Seated Posture and Alignment

To attain optimal seated posture and alignment in Chair Pilates, follow these guidelines:

1. Start with a Stable Base: Begin by positioning your chair on a stable surface, ensuring that all chair legs are in contact with the floor.

2. Sitting Bones: When sitting on the chair, find your sitting bones (ischial tuberosities), which are the bony protrusions at the base of your pelvis. Position them evenly on the chair seat.

3. Neutral Pelvis: Maintain a neutral pelvis, which means that your pelvis is neither tilted forward nor backward. This position aligns the natural curves of your spine and supports proper posture.

4. Engage Your Core: Initiate core engagement by drawing your navel slightly inward and upward toward your spine.

This action stabilizes your core and provides support for your back.

5. Straight Back: Sit with a straight back and an elongated spine. Imagine a string pulling you upward from the top of your head. This visualization encourages a tall and lifted posture.

6. Shoulder Placement: Roll your shoulders back and down, avoiding tension in the neck and upper traps. Your shoulder blades should move toward each other slightly to create a broad chest.

7. Chest Lift: Lift your chest while maintaining a natural, relaxed curve in your lower back. Avoid overarching or rounding the spine excessively.

8. Head Position: Keep your head in line with your spine, looking straight ahead. Avoid jutting your chin forward or tilting your head down.

9. Relaxed Arms and Hands: Your arms should be relaxed by your sides, and your hands can rest lightly on the chair handles or your lap.

10. Even Weight Distribution: Ensure that your weight is evenly distributed between both sitting bones, avoiding favoring one side over the other.

11. Breathing: Practice controlled and mindful breathing. Inhale deeply into your diaphragm, allowing your ribcage to expand, and exhale fully. Coordinating your breath with your seated posture enhances core engagement and relaxation.

Maintaining Seated Posture and Alignment during Exercises

During Chair Pilates exercises, it's essential to maintain your seated posture and alignment. Here are a few additional considerations:

- Focus on your core engagement to provide stability and support during movements.
- Continue to breathe mindfully, coordinating your breath with each exercise.
- Pay attention to the specific cues and guidance provided by your Chair Pilates instructor or guide for each exercise.

By consistently applying these principles of seated posture and alignment, you can achieve a solid foundation for your Chair Pilates practice. This foundational knowledge will help you perform exercises safely and effectively while promoting overall well-being and body awareness.

Breathing Techniques

Breathing is a fundamental element of Chair Pilates, as it plays a vital role in enhancing the effectiveness and mindfulness of your practice. The right breathing techniques in Chair Pilates not only facilitate the flow of oxygen to your muscles but also promote relaxation, focus, and control during exercises. This exploration will delve into the importance of proper breathing techniques in Chair Pilates and provide guidance on how to coordinate your breath with your movements.

The Importance of Breath in Chair Pilates

In Chair Pilates, controlled and mindful breathing is integral to the practice for several reasons:

1. Oxygenation of Muscles: Efficient breathing ensures that your muscles receive an optimal supply of oxygen, enhancing endurance and performance during exercises.

2. Core Engagement: Proper breathing is closely tied to core engagement. Coordinating your breath with movements can help activate the core muscles, enhancing stability and control.

3. Stress Reduction: The controlled breathing techniques in Chair Pilates promote relaxation and reduce stress. Mindful breath work encourages a sense of calm and focus, reducing anxiety and tension.

4. Mind-Body Connection: Chair Pilates places a strong emphasis on the mind-body connection. Coordinated breathing fosters this connection, making you more aware of your body's movements and positioning.

Breathing Techniques in Chair Pilates

Chair Pilates utilizes specific breathing techniques that vary depending on the type of exercise and its intended effect. Here are the two primary breathing techniques employed in Chair Pilates:

1. Lateral Breathing:

- Lateral breathing is the most common breathing technique in Chair Pilates. It involves inhaling through the nose and allowing the breath to expand the ribcage laterally (out to the sides) and into the back. This type of breath is deep and diaphragmatic, filling the lower lungs and promoting core engagement.

- Lateral breathing is typically used during exercises that require core stability, such as when performing abdominal exercises, seated leg lifts, or arm movements.

2. Thoracic Breathing:

- Thoracic breathing involves inhaling through the nose and allowing the breath to expand the ribcage upward and forward. This type of breath is employed during exercises that require spinal flexibility, such as those targeting the upper back and shoulders.
- Thoracic breathing can help open the chest and enhance the mobility of the thoracic spine, but it is typically reserved for specific exercises that focus on the upper body.

Breathing Guidelines for Chair Pilates

To incorporate proper breathing techniques into your Chair Pilates practice, follow these guidelines:

1. Start with Diaphragmatic Breathing: Before you begin your exercises, engage in diaphragmatic breathing. Inhale deeply through your nose, expanding your abdomen, and then exhale slowly through your mouth.

This practice can help you relax and prepare for your Chair Pilates session.

2. Lateral Breathing for Stability: Use lateral breathing during exercises that require core stability and engagement. Inhale through your nose, allowing your ribcage to expand laterally.

As you exhale through your mouth, draw your navel slightly inward and upward to engage the core.

3. Thoracic Breathing for Flexibility: Employ thoracic breathing during exercises that focus on spinal flexibility and upper body movements. Inhale through your nose, allowing your ribcage to expand upward and forward.

As you exhale through your mouth, maintain this expansion to encourage thoracic mobility.

4. Coordinate with Movements: Sync your breath with your movements. Inhale as you prepare for a movement, and exhale as you execute it. For example, during a seated leg lift, you would inhale as you prepare and exhale as you lift your leg.

5. Stay Mindful: Be present and mindful of your breath throughout your practice. Use your breath as a tool to maintain control, stability, and relaxation during each exercise.

Breath as a Guiding Force in Chair Pilates

Breathing techniques in Chair Pilates serve as a guiding force, enhancing your practice's effectiveness and depth.

Proper breathing techniques facilitate core engagement, promote relaxation, and encourage a strong mind-body connection.

By incorporating the principles of lateral and thoracic breathing and coordinating your breath with your movements, you can enrich your Chair Pilates experience and enjoy the numerous physical and mental benefits it offers.

Warm-up Exercises

A well-executed warm-up is a crucial component of any fitness routine, including Chair Pilates. A proper warm-up prepares your body for more intense movements, reduces the risk of injury, and enhances the effectiveness of your exercises.

In Chair Pilates, warm-up exercises are essential to activate core muscles, improve circulation, and establish the mind-body connection. This guide will introduce you to key warm-up exercises for Chair Pilates and explain their significance in your practice.

Importance of Warm-up Exercises in Chair Pilates

1. Muscle Activation: A warm-up increases blood flow to your muscles, which helps activate them for subsequent exercises. This prepares your body to engage core muscles effectively during Chair Pilates movements.

2. Flexibility and Mobility: Warm-up exercises improve joint flexibility and range of motion, making it easier to perform Chair Pilates exercises that require controlled movements and proper alignment.

3. Injury Prevention: A thorough warm-up reduces the risk of injury by preparing your muscles and joints for the demands of Chair Pilates. It helps to prevent strains, sprains, and muscle imbalances.

4. Mind-Body Connection: Warm-up exercises provide an opportunity to establish a mind-body connection, allowing you to focus on your breath, posture, and alignment, setting a mindful tone for the rest of your practice.

Warm-up Exercises for Chair Pilates

Here are some effective warm-up exercises to incorporate into your Chair Pilates routine:

1. Seated Marching: Sit at the edge of your chair with a straight back. Lift one knee towards your chest, then lower it and alternate with the other knee. This exercise warms up your hip flexors and improves circulation.

2. Shoulder Rolls: Sit with your feet flat on the floor and your arms relaxed by your sides. Inhale, and as you exhale, roll your shoulders back and down in a circular motion. This exercise loosens up the shoulder joints and relieves tension.

3. Neck Tilts: Sit up tall with your feet flat. Gently tilt your head to the right, bringing your right ear towards your right shoulder. Hold for a few seconds, then switch to the left side. This exercise releases tension in the neck and upper back.

4. Pelvic Tilts: Sit with your feet flat and your hands on your knees. Inhale, and as you exhale, tuck your pelvis under, rounding your lower back. Then inhale, arch your lower back, and tilt your pelvis forward. Repeat this motion a few times to warm up your lower back and hips.

5. Ankle Pumps: Sit with your feet flat and extend your legs. Flex and point your toes, alternating between the two movements. This exercise enhances circulation in the lower legs and feet.

6. Seated Spinal Twist: Sit with your feet flat and your hands on your knees. Inhale, then exhale as you twist your upper body to the right, bringing your left hand to your right knee and your right hand behind you. Inhale to return to the center, then repeat on the left side. This exercise mobilizes the spine and enhances torso flexibility.

7. Diaphragmatic Breathing: Sit with a straight back. Place one hand on your chest and the other on your abdomen. Inhale deeply through your nose, allowing your abdomen to rise and your diaphragm to engage. Exhale slowly through your mouth. This exercise establishes a mindful breath pattern for your practice.

Perform these warm-up exercises at the beginning of your Chair Pilates session, dedicating 5-10 minutes to prepare your body for the main exercises. Focus on your breath and alignment during the warm-up, setting the tone for a mindful and controlled practice.

By incorporating these warm-up exercises, you'll enhance the safety and effectiveness of your Chair Pilates routine, ensuring that your body is adequately prepared for the challenges and benefits that Chair Pilates has to offer.

Core Strengthening Exercises

A strong and stable core is at the heart of Chair Pilates, and core strengthening exercises play a central role in this practice. The chair apparatus provides a versatile platform for targeting the muscles of your core, including the abdominals, lower back, and pelvic floor.

A well-developed core not only enhances your posture and balance but also supports the execution of more complex Chair Pilates movements. In this guide, we will explore key core strengthening exercises in Chair Pilates and their significance in achieving a strong and stable core.

Importance of Core Strengthening in Chair Pilates

1. Core Stability: A strong core provides stability and support for your spine and pelvis, reducing the risk of back pain and improving overall posture.

2. Enhanced Balance: Core strength is essential for maintaining balance and stability during Chair Pilates exercises, particularly those that involve lifting and extending the legs.

3. Improved Posture: A strong core helps you maintain an upright and aligned posture, reducing the risk of slouching and associated discomfort.

4. Optimal Movement: Core strengthening exercises are essential for executing Chair Pilates movements with precision and control. A strong core allows for fluid and controlled movements, enhancing the effectiveness of your practice.

Core Strengthening Exercises in Chair Pilates

1. Seated Spine Stretch: Sit at the edge of the chair with your feet flat on the floor. Extend your arms forward at shoulder height. Inhale to lengthen your spine, and exhale to round your spine, reaching your fingertips toward your toes. Inhale to return to an upright position. This exercise targets the entire spine, improving flexibility and core engagement.

2. Single-Leg Lifts: Sit with your feet flat on the floor. Extend one leg straight while lifting it off the floor, keeping the core engaged. Hold for a moment and lower it back down. Alternate legs. This exercise challenges the lower abdominal muscles and improves leg strength and balance.

3. Twisting Abdominal Toner: Sit up tall and hold the chair handles. Inhale, and as you exhale, twist your upper body to one side, engaging your oblique muscles. Inhale to return to the center and exhale to twist to the other side. This exercise targets the obliques and enhances core stability.

4. Chair Teaser: Sit on the edge of the chair with your feet off the ground and knees bent. Hold the chair handles for support. Inhale, and as you exhale, extend your legs forward and lean your upper body back. Inhale to return to the starting position. This exercise challenges the entire core and enhances balance.

5. Chair Roll-Ups: Sit at the edge of the chair with your legs extended and feet flexed. Inhale, and as you exhale, round your spine and roll down, reaching your hands toward your feet. Inhale to return to an upright position. This exercise strengthens the entire core and improves flexibility.

6. Pelvic Lifts: Sit with your feet flat on the floor and hands resting on the chair handles. Inhale, and as you exhale, lift your hips off the chair while engaging your glutes and core. Inhale to lower your hips. This exercise targets the lower back, glutes, and hamstrings, enhancing core stability.

7. Footwork Variations: Perform various footwork exercises on the chair, such as heel raises, toe raises, and circles. These movements engage the leg muscles and core, promoting balance and strength.

8. Hundred Prep: Sit with your feet flat on the floor and hold the chair handles. Inhale, and as you exhale, lift your feet off the ground, engaging your core. Pump your arms up and down as you inhale for five counts and exhale for five counts. This exercise challenges the core and enhances control.

Perform these core strengthening exercises regularly to build a strong and stable core foundation for your Chair Pilates practice.

Focus on proper alignment and controlled movements to maximize the benefits and minimize the risk of injury.

Upper Body Exercises

While Chair Pilates is renowned for its core-strengthening benefits, it also offers a range of upper body exercises that promote strength, flexibility, and improved posture.

These exercises target the muscles of the upper back, shoulders, arms, and chest.

In addition to building upper body strength, these movements enhance overall body balance and alignment, making Chair Pilates a comprehensive workout. This guide explores key upper body exercises in Chair Pilates and their significance in achieving upper body strength and flexibility.

Importance of Upper Body Exercises in Chair Pilates

1. Improved Posture: Upper body exercises in Chair Pilates help counter the effects of prolonged sitting and screen time, promoting an open chest and a balanced, upright posture.

2. Upper Body Strength: These exercises target the muscles of the upper back, shoulders, arms, and chest, enhancing strength and toning.

3. Enhanced Flexibility: Upper body exercises encourage greater flexibility in the shoulder joints and upper spine, which can alleviate tension and improve range of motion.

4. Balanced Development: Combining core and upper body exercises creates a holistic approach to fitness, reducing the risk of muscle imbalances and postural issues.

Upper Body Exercises in Chair Pilates

1. Shoulder Rolls: Sit with your feet flat on the floor. Inhale, and as you exhale, roll your shoulders back and down in a circular motion. This exercise loosens up the shoulder joints and relieves tension.

2. Arm Circles: Sit with your feet flat and your arms extended to the sides. Inhale, and as you exhale, make small forward circles with your arms. Reverse the direction of the circles after several repetitions. This exercise enhances shoulder flexibility and stability.

3. Chest Expansion: Sit with your feet flat and hold the chair handles. Inhale, and as you exhale, extend your arms back, opening your chest and shoulders. Inhale to return to the starting position.

This exercise targets the chest and shoulder muscles, promoting upper body strength and flexibility.

4. Lateral Arm Raises: Sit with your feet flat and your arms relaxed by your sides. Inhale, and as you exhale, raise your arms to the sides at shoulder level. Inhale to lower your arms. This exercise enhances the strength of the shoulder muscles.

5. Seated Tricep Dips: Sit at the edge of the chair with your feet flat and hands on the chair seat beside your hips. Inhale, and as you exhale, lift your hips off the chair, straightening your arms. Inhale to lower your hips. This exercise targets the triceps and enhances arm strength.

6. Bicep Curls: Sit with your feet flat and arms by your sides. Hold light hand weights (if available). Inhale, and as you exhale, curl your arms upward to bring the weights toward your shoulders. Inhale to lower the weights. This exercise strengthens the biceps.

7. Spine Stretch: Sit with your feet flat and legs extended. Inhale, and as you exhale, round your spine and reach your arms forward, stretching your upper back and shoulders. Inhale to return to an upright position. This exercise enhances upper body flexibility and posture.

8. Swan Dive: Sit with your feet flat and arms extended forward. Inhale, and as you exhale, lift your arms and upper body off the chair while keeping your feet on the ground. Inhale to lower your body. This exercise targets the upper back and shoulder muscles.

By incorporating these upper body exercises into your Chair Pilates routine, you can achieve a more balanced and toned upper body, alleviate tension, and promote better posture. Focus on proper alignment, controlled movements, and proper breathing to maximize the benefits of these exercises.

Lower Body Exercises

Lower body exercises in Chair Pilates are essential for targeting the muscles of the legs, hips, and buttocks. These movements promote strength, flexibility, and balance in the lower body while also supporting overall posture and alignment.

By incorporating lower body exercises into your Chair Pilates routine, you can achieve a comprehensive full-body workout. This guide explores key lower body exercises in Chair Pilates and their significance in building lower body strength and flexibility.

Importance of Lower Body Exercises in Chair Pilates

1. Lower Body Strength: These exercises focus on the muscles of the legs, including the quadriceps, hamstrings, calves, and glutes, enhancing strength and toning.

2. Balance and Stability: Lower body exercises in Chair Pilates challenge balance and stability, promoting better control during various movements.

3. Increased Flexibility: These movements encourage greater flexibility in the hips, knees, and ankles, improving overall range of motion.

4. Alignment and Posture: By strengthening the lower body, you can better support your spine's natural curvature, which contributes to better posture and reduced lower back strain.

Lower Body Exercises in Chair Pilates

1. Chair Squats: Sit at the edge of the chair with your feet hip-width apart. Inhale, and as you exhale, stand up from the chair, extending your hips and knees. Inhale to sit back down. This exercise targets the quadriceps, hamstrings, and glutes, promoting lower body strength.

2. Leg Lifts: Sit with your feet flat on the floor and hold the chair handles. Inhale, and as you exhale, lift one leg straight in front of you. Inhale to lower the leg. Repeat on the other side. This exercise targets the quadriceps and hip flexors, improving leg strength and balance.

3. Seated Leg Circles: Sit with your feet flat on the floor. Extend one leg and make small circles with your foot. Reverse the direction of the circles after several repetitions. This exercise enhances ankle mobility and works the quadriceps and hip muscles.

4. Seated Inner Thigh Squeeze: Sit with your feet flat on the floor and a ball or cushion between your knees. Inhale, and as you exhale, squeeze the ball with your knees. Inhale to release. This exercise targets the inner thigh muscles, promoting leg strength and alignment.

5. Calf Raises: Sit with your feet flat on the floor. Inhale, and as you exhale, lift your heels off the ground, engaging your calf muscles. Inhale to lower your heels. This exercise strengthens the calf muscles and improves ankle stability.

6. Footwork Variations Perform various footwork exercises on the chair, such as heel raises, toe raises, and circles. These movements engage the leg muscles, promoting balance and strength.

7. Single-Leg Extensions: Sit with your feet flat on the floor. Inhale, and as you exhale, extend one leg straight while keeping the core engaged. Hold for a moment and lower it back down. Repeat on the other side. This exercise challenges the quadriceps and enhances leg strength and balance.

8. Pelvic Lifts: Sit with your feet flat on the floor and hands resting on the chair handles. Inhale, and as you exhale, lift your hips off the chair while engaging your glutes and core. Inhale to lower your hips.

This exercise targets the lower back, glutes, and hamstrings, promoting lower body stability.

By incorporating these lower body exercises into your Chair Pilates routine, you can achieve a well-rounded lower body workout, improve strength and flexibility, and enhance balance and stability.

Focus on proper alignment, controlled movements, and proper breathing to maximize the benefits of these exercises.

Cool-down Stretches

Cool-down stretches are an essential part of your Chair Pilates routine. After an invigorating workout, they help you relax, increase flexibility, and promote recovery.

These stretches target the muscles that have been engaged during your practice, allowing them to elongate and reduce tension.

Incorporating cool-down stretches into your Chair Pilates routine can enhance your flexibility, prevent muscle soreness, and provide a sense of relaxation.

This guide explores key cool-down stretches in Chair Pilates and their importance in your post-workout routine.

Importance of Cool-Down Stretches in Chair Pilates

1. Muscle Relaxation: Cool-down stretches help to reduce muscle tension and promote relaxation after an intense workout.

2. Flexibility: These stretches enhance muscle flexibility and joint range of motion, making it easier to achieve proper posture and alignment.

3. Injury Prevention: Stretching after exercise reduces the risk of muscle strains and imbalances, contributing to injury prevention.

4. Mind-Body Connection: Cool-down stretches provide an opportunity to center yourself, focus on your breath, and maintain the mind-body connection cultivated during your practice.

Cool-Down Stretches in Chair Pilates

1. Seated Forward Bend: Sit on the edge of the chair with your feet flat on the floor. Inhale, lengthen your spine, and exhale as you fold forward from your hips. Reach your hands toward your feet. Hold the stretch for 20-30 seconds. This stretch targets the hamstrings and lower back.

2. Seated Spinal Twist: Sit at the edge of the chair with your feet flat. Inhale, and as you exhale, twist your upper body to one side, bringing your opposite hand to the outside of your knee. Hold for 20-30 seconds, then switch sides. This stretch improves spinal mobility and relieves tension in the back and shoulders.

3. Chest Opener: Sit with your feet flat and hold the chair handles behind you. Inhale, and as you exhale, gently lift your chest and open your shoulders. Hold for 20-30 seconds. This stretch relieves tension in the chest and shoulders.

4. Seated Quad Stretch: Sit with your feet flat on the floor. Inhale, and as you exhale, lift one foot and bring it toward your glutes. Hold your ankle or foot with one hand to stretch the quadriceps. Hold for 20-30 seconds, then switch legs.

5. Seated Hip Flexor Stretch: Sit with one foot flat on the floor and extend the other leg straight. Inhale, and as you exhale, lean forward slightly to stretch the hip flexor of the extended leg. Hold for 20-30 seconds, then switch legs.

6. Inner Thigh Stretch: Sit with your feet flat and place the soles of your feet together. Hold your feet with your hands.

Inhale, and as you exhale, gently press your knees toward the floor to stretch the inner thighs. Hold for 20-30 seconds.

7. Ankle Stretch: Sit with your feet flat and extend one leg straight. Point and flex your toes several times to stretch the ankle. Repeat with the other leg.

8. Diaphragmatic Breathing: Finish your cool-down with a few deep diaphragmatic breaths. Inhale deeply through your nose, expanding your abdomen, and exhale slowly through your mouth.

This brings a sense of relaxation and mindfulness to your post-workout routine.

Perform these cool-down stretches after your Chair Pilates workout to relax, enhance flexibility, and promote muscle recovery. Hold each stretch for 20-30 seconds, and breathe deeply to facilitate relaxation and the release of tension.

CHAPTER THREE

Chair Pilates Routines for Beginners

Chair Pilates, a modification of the classical Pilates method, offers an accessible and effective way to develop strength, flexibility, and overall wellness.

Designed with the beginner in mind, Chair Pilates routines provide a gentle introduction to the principles and exercises of Pilates, all while utilizing a chair as the primary piece of equipment. Whether you're new to exercise or looking to diversify your fitness regimen, Chair Pilates is an excellent choice to embark on a journey of physical and mental transformation.

The Essence of Chair Pilates

Pilates, originally developed by Joseph Pilates in the early 20th century, is renowned for its focus on core strength, flexibility, balance, and improved posture.

While traditional Pilates often employs specialized equipment like the reformer, cadillac, and mat, Chair Pilates simplifies the method by incorporating a chair, making it more approachable for individuals of all fitness levels.

The chair provides support and stability, allowing beginners to comfortably perform a wide range of Pilates exercises while emphasizing proper alignment and controlled movements.

The Appeal of Chair Pilates for Beginners

Chair Pilates appeals to beginners for several compelling reasons:

1. Accessibility: The chair is a common piece of furniture found in homes, which makes Chair Pilates an affordable and accessible exercise option. You don't need access to a **fully equipped Pilates studio to begin your practice.**

2. Gentle Introduction: Chair Pilates routines are designed to be gentle on the body, making it suitable for those who may be new to exercise or have physical limitations. It provides a controlled and low-impact environment for learning Pilates principles.

3. Core Emphasis: Chair Pilates places a strong emphasis on core strength, which is foundational for overall wellness and functional movement. The chair offers support and guidance for developing a strong core.

4. Improved Posture: Many beginners seek to enhance their posture, especially in a world where prolonged sitting and screen time are prevalent. Chair Pilates promotes an upright and aligned posture, reducing the risk of discomfort and injury.

5. Mind-Body Connection: Chair Pilates encourages a strong mind-body connection. Beginners can learn to be more mindful of their movements, breath, and alignment, fostering greater awareness of their bodies.

6. Customizable Workouts: Chair Pilates routines can be customized to suit individual fitness levels. As beginners progress, they can gradually increase the intensity and complexity of their workouts.

Building a Foundation in Chair Pilates

For beginners, it's essential to establish a strong foundation in Chair Pilates. This begins with understanding the core principles of Pilates, including concentration, control, centering, precision, and breath. Chair Pilates routines guide beginners through the process of mastering these principles and gradually introduce exercises that align with their skill level.

Key elements of building a foundation in Chair Pilates include:

1. Proper Alignment: Learning how to sit and position yourself on the chair to maintain proper alignment of the spine, pelvis, and limbs. Proper alignment is fundamental to the safety and effectiveness of Chair Pilates.

2. Controlled Movements: Chair Pilates emphasizes controlled, precise movements. Beginners focus on moving with intention and control, ensuring each exercise is executed mindfully.

3. Breath Awareness: Breath awareness is vital in Chair Pilates, and beginners are introduced to coordinated breathing techniques that enhance core engagement and relaxation.

4. Foundational Exercises: Chair Pilates for beginners includes a series of foundational exercises that build strength and flexibility. These exercises are designed to be accessible and progressively challenging.

5. Safety and Alignment: Safety considerations are a top priority for beginners. Chair Pilates routines teach proper alignment and techniques to minimize the risk of injury and strain.

6. Progressive Workouts: As beginners become more confident and proficient, Chair Pilates routines offer opportunities to progress and take on more advanced exercises while maintaining an appropriate level of challenge.

Embrace the Journey

Embarking on a Chair Pilates journey as a beginner is an invitation to discover the benefits of this well-rounded practice. From enhancing physical strength and flexibility to fostering a deep connection between body and mind, Chair Pilates is an enriching experience that supports overall wellness.

By building a strong foundation and gradually advancing your skills, you can unlock the transformative power of Chair Pilates in your life. The chair becomes not just a piece of furniture but a valuable tool in your pursuit of health and vitality.

As you embrace this journey, Chair Pilates has the potential to lead you to newfound levels of well-being and fitness.

Morning Chair Pilates Routine

A morning Chair Pilates routine is a fantastic way to kickstart your day with energy, vitality, and a sense of well-being.

This routine is designed to be gentle, making it an ideal choice for your morning workout, especially if you're a beginner or looking for a low-impact, accessible exercise routine. Chair Pilates in the morning can help you improve posture, boost your energy levels, and prepare your body and mind for the day ahead. Let's get started!

Preparation:

- Place a sturdy chair in a quiet and spacious area.
- Wear comfortable workout attire.
- Begin with diaphragmatic breathing to center yourself. Inhale deeply through your nose, expanding your abdomen, and exhale slowly through your mouth.

1. Seated Marching (2 minutes):

- Sit on the edge of the chair with your feet flat on the floor.

- Lift one knee toward your chest, then lower it.

- Alternate legs in a controlled and rhythmic manner.

2. Arm Circles (1 minute):

- Sit with your feet flat and arms extended to the sides.

- Inhale, and as you exhale, make small forward circles with your arms.

- After 30 seconds, reverse the direction of the circles.

3. Seated Spinal Twist (1 minute):

- Sit with your feet flat and hands on your knees.

- Inhale, and as you exhale, twist your upper body to one side.

- Inhale to return to the center, then exhale and twist to the other side.

4. Chest Expansion (1 minute):

- Sit with your feet flat and hold the chair handles.

- Inhale, and as you exhale, gently extend your arms back, opening your chest.

- Inhale to return to the starting position.

5. Seated Quad Stretch (1 minute):

- Sit with your feet flat on the floor.
- Inhale, and as you exhale, lift one foot and bring it toward your glutes.
- Hold your ankle or foot with one hand to stretch the quadriceps.
- Hold for 30 seconds, then switch legs.

6. Chair Squats (2 minutes):

- Sit on the edge of the chair with your feet hip-width apart.
- Inhale, and as you exhale, stand up from the chair, extending your hips and knees.
- Inhale to sit back down.

7. Seated Forward Bend (1 minute):

- Sit on the edge of the chair with your feet flat on the floor.
- Inhale to lengthen your spine, and exhale as you fold forward from your hips.
- Reach your hands toward your feet.

8. Diaphragmatic Breathing (2 minutes): Finish your morning routine with a few deep diaphragmatic breaths. Inhale deeply through your nose, expanding your abdomen, and exhale slowly through your mouth. Focus on your breath and a sense of relaxation.

Midday Energy Booster

Feeling a midday slump? Chair Pilates to the rescue! This energizing routine is designed to rejuvenate your body and mind during that midday lull. It's a quick and effective way to boost your energy, improve your focus, and revitalize your posture. Best of all, it can be done right at your desk or in a quiet corner. Let's get started with this short and invigorating Chair Pilates routine.

Preparation:

- Find a quiet and comfortable space where you won't be interrupted.
- Sit on a sturdy chair with your feet flat on the floor.
- Take a few moments for diaphragmatic breathing to center yourself. Inhale deeply through your nose, expanding your abdomen, and exhale slowly through your mouth.

1. Seated Marching (1 minute):

- Sit at the edge of the chair with your feet flat on the floor.
- Lift one knee toward your chest, then lower it.
- Alternate legs in a controlled and rhythmic manner.

2. Arm Circles (1 minute):

- Sit with your feet flat and arms extended to the sides.
- Inhale, and as you exhale, make small forward circles with your arms.
- After 30 seconds, reverse the direction of the circles.

3. Seated Spinal Twist (1 minute):

- Sit with your feet flat and hands on your knees.
- Inhale, and as you exhale, twist your upper body to one side.
- Inhale to return to the center, then exhale and twist to the other side.

4. Chest Expansion (1 minute):

- Sit with your feet flat and hold the chair handles.
- Inhale, and as you exhale, gently extend your arms back, opening your chest.

- Inhale to return to the starting position.

5. Seated Quad Stretch (1 minute):

- Sit with your feet flat on the floor.
- Inhale, and as you exhale, lift one foot and bring it toward your glutes.
- Hold your ankle or foot with one hand to stretch the quadriceps.
- Hold for 30 seconds, then switch legs.

6. Chair Squats (2 minutes):

- Sit on the edge of the chair with your feet hip-width apart.
- Inhale, and as you exhale, stand up from the chair, extending your hips and knees.
- Inhale to sit back down.

7. Seated Forward Bend (1 minute):

- Sit on the edge of the chair with your feet flat on the floor.
- Inhale to lengthen your spine, and exhale as you fold forward from your hips.
- Reach your hands toward your feet.

8. Diaphragmatic Breathing (2 minutes): Finish your midday routine with a few deep diaphragmatic breaths. Inhale deeply through your nose, expanding your abdomen, and exhale slowly through your mouth. Focus on your breath and a sense of revitalization.

Evening Relaxation Sequence

As the day winds down, it's essential to unwind and find relaxation. Chair Pilates can offer a perfect way to release tension and promote a sense of tranquility.

This evening relaxation sequence is designed to help you transition from the busyness of the day to a peaceful and restful evening. With gentle exercises and mindful breathing, you can create a sense of calm and well-being. Let's begin this soothing Chair Pilates sequence.

Preparation:

- Find a quiet and calming space free from distractions.
- Sit on a sturdy chair with your feet flat on the floor.
- Start with diaphragmatic breathing to calm your mind. Inhale deeply through your nose, expanding

your abdomen, and exhale slowly through your mouth.

1. Seated Marching (2 minutes):

- Sit on the edge of the chair with your feet flat on the floor.
- Lift one knee toward your chest, then lower it.
- Alternate legs in a controlled and rhythmic manner.

2. Arm Circles (2 minutes):

- Sit with your feet flat and arms extended to the sides.
- Inhale, and as you exhale, make small forward circles with your arms.
- After 1 minute, reverse the direction of the circles.

3. Seated Spinal Twist (2 minutes):

- Sit with your feet flat and hands on your knees.
- Inhale, and as you exhale, twist your upper body to one side.
- Inhale to return to the center, then exhale and twist to the other side.

4. Chest Expansion (2 minutes):

- Sit with your feet flat and hold the chair handles.
- Inhale, and as you exhale, gently extend your arms back, opening your chest.
- Inhale to return to the starting position.

5. Seated Quad Stretch (2 minutes):

- Sit with your feet flat on the floor.
- Inhale, and as you exhale, lift one foot and bring it toward your glutes.
- Hold your ankle or foot with one hand to stretch the quadriceps.
- Hold for 1 minute, then switch legs.

6. Chair Squats (3 minutes):

- Sit on the edge of the chair with your feet hip-width apart.
- Inhale, and as you exhale, stand up from the chair, extending your hips and knees.
- Inhale to sit back down.

7. Seated Forward Bend (2 minutes):

- Sit on the edge of the chair with your feet flat on the floor.
- Inhale to lengthen your spine, and exhale as you fold forward from your hips.
- Reach your hands toward your feet.

8. Diaphragmatic Breathing and Mindfulness (3 minutes): Finish your evening relaxation sequence with diaphragmatic breathing. Inhale deeply through your nose, expanding your abdomen, and exhale slowly through your mouth. Focus on your breath and bring your awareness to the present moment.

Chair Pilates for Posture Improvement

Poor posture is a common issue in our modern, sedentary lifestyles. Chair Pilates offers an effective and accessible way to address this problem, helping you build the core strength, flexibility, and awareness needed to improve your posture.

This Chair Pilates routine focuses on exercises that target the muscles responsible for maintaining good posture.

By integrating these exercises into your routine, you can gradually create lasting improvements in your posture.

Preparation:

- Choose a sturdy chair and find a quiet space where you can focus on your practice.
- Wear comfortable clothing that allows for a full range of motion.
- Start with diaphragmatic breathing to center yourself. Inhale deeply through your nose, expanding your abdomen, and exhale slowly through your mouth.

1. Seated Marching (2 minutes):

- Sit on the edge of the chair with your feet flat on the floor.
- Lift one knee toward your chest, then lower it.
- Alternate legs in a controlled and rhythmic manner.
- This exercise engages the core and hip flexors, helping to relieve lower back strain.

2. Seated Spinal Twist (2 minutes):

- Sit with your feet flat on the floor and hands on your knees.
- Inhale, and as you exhale, twist your upper body to one side.
- Inhale to return to the center, then exhale and twist to the other side.
- This exercise enhances spinal mobility and opens the chest.

3. Chest Expansion (2 minutes):

- Sit with your feet flat and hold the chair handles.
- Inhale, and as you exhale, gently extend your arms back, opening your chest.
- Inhale to return to the starting position.
- This exercise strengthens the upper back and shoulders, which are crucial for supporting an upright posture.

4. Seated Quad Stretch (2 minutes):

- Sit with your feet flat on the floor.
- Inhale, and as you exhale, lift one foot and bring it toward your glutes.

- Hold your ankle or foot with one hand to stretch the quadriceps.
- Hold for 1 minute, then switch legs.
- Stretching the quadriceps helps alleviate tension in the front of the hips, promoting a balanced pelvis.

5. Chair Squats (3 minutes):

- Sit on the edge of the chair with your feet hip-width apart.
- Inhale, and as you exhale, stand up from the chair, extending your hips and knees.
- Inhale to sit back down.
- Chair squats strengthen the glutes, hamstrings, and quadriceps, which are key for supporting an upright posture.

6. Seated Forward Bend (2 minutes):

- Sit on the edge of the chair with your feet flat on the floor.
- Inhale to lengthen your spine, and exhale as you fold forward from your hips.
- Reach your hands toward your feet.

- This exercise stretches the hamstrings and promotes spinal flexibility.

7. Diaphragmatic Breathing and Mindfulness (3 minutes):

- Finish your routine with diaphragmatic breathing, focusing on your breath and mindfulness.
- Inhale deeply through your nose, expanding your abdomen, and exhale slowly through your mouth.

Chair Pilates for Stress Relief

Chair Pilates can be a wonderful way to relieve stress, relax both your body and mind, and find a sense of calm and tranquility.

This Chair Pilates routine is designed to help you de-stress, release tension, and improve your overall well-being. It's a gentle practice that can be performed in a chair, making it accessible and convenient.

Whether you've had a long day or just need a moment to unwind, this routine can help you find relief from stress.

Preparation:

- Find a quiet and comfortable space where you won't be disturbed.
- Sit on a sturdy chair with your feet flat on the floor.
- Begin with diaphragmatic breathing to center yourself. Inhale deeply through your nose, expanding your abdomen, and exhale slowly through your mouth.

1. Seated Marching (2 minutes):

- Sit on the edge of the chair with your feet flat on the floor.
- Lift one knee toward your chest, then lower it.
- Alternate legs in a controlled and rhythmic manner.

2. Arm Circles (2 minutes):

- Sit with your feet flat and arms extended to the sides.
- Inhale, and as you exhale, make small forward circles with your arms.
- After 1 minute, reverse the direction of the circles.

3. Seated Spinal Twist (2 minutes):

- Sit with your feet flat on the floor and hands on your knees.
- Inhale, and as you exhale, twist your upper body to one side.
- Inhale to return to the center, then exhale and twist to the other side.

4. Chest Expansion (2 minutes):

- Sit with your feet flat and hold the chair handles.
- Inhale, and as you exhale, gently extend your arms back, opening your chest.
- Inhale to return to the starting position.

5. Seated Quad Stretch (2 minutes):

- Sit with your feet flat on the floor.
- Inhale, and as you exhale, lift one foot and bring it toward your glutes.
- Hold your ankle or foot with one hand to stretch the quadriceps.
- Hold for 1 minute, then switch legs.

6. Chair Squats (3 minutes):

- Sit on the edge of the chair with your feet hip-width apart.
- Inhale, and as you exhale, stand up from the chair, extending your hips and knees.
- Inhale to sit back down.

7. Seated Forward Bend (2 minutes):

- Sit on the edge of the chair with your feet flat on the floor.
- Inhale to lengthen your spine, and exhale as you fold forward from your hips.
- Reach your hands toward your feet.

8. Diaphragmatic Breathing and Mindfulness (3 minutes):

- Finish your stress relief routine with diaphragmatic breathing and mindfulness.
- Inhale deeply through your nose, expanding your abdomen, and exhale slowly through your mouth.
- Focus on your breath and bring your awareness to the present moment.

CHAPTER FOUR

Chair Pilates for Wellness

In an era marked by increasingly sedentary lifestyles and the pressures of modern living, the pursuit of wellness has become a paramount goal for many. Wellness encompasses not only physical health but also mental and emotional well-being. As individuals seek holistic approaches to enhance their quality of life, Chair Pilates emerges as a versatile and effective method for promoting wellness.

This comprehensive introduction delves into the world of Chair Pilates, exploring its principles, benefits, and applications in the pursuit of holistic wellness.

The Essence of Chair Pilates

Pilates, a method developed by Joseph Pilates in the early 20th century, has long been revered for its holistic approach to health and fitness.

While traditional Pilates often involves specialized equipment and mat exercises, Chair Pilates simplifies the method by utilizing a common chair as the primary apparatus. This modification makes Pilates accessible to individuals of all fitness levels, including those who may have physical limitations or require a gentle and supportive entry into the world of exercise.

Chair Pilates adheres to the foundational principles of Pilates, which include concentration, control, centering, precision, and breath. By focusing on these principles, Chair Pilates nurtures the body-mind connection, emphasizing the importance of mindfulness in each movement. As a result, this practice extends beyond physical exercise, fostering a sense of mental clarity and emotional balance, which are integral components of overall wellness.

Key Components of Chair Pilates for Wellness

1. Physical Fitness: Chair Pilates provides a well-rounded approach to physical fitness. It focuses on core strength, flexibility, balance, and posture. These elements are pivotal in promoting the physical aspect of wellness, as they help maintain a healthy body and prevent musculoskeletal issues.

2. Mental Clarity: The emphasis on concentration and mindfulness in Chair Pilates cultivates mental clarity and cognitive well-being. The practice encourages you to stay present, enhancing your ability to manage stress and reduce anxiety.

3. Emotional Balance: Chair Pilates offers a sanctuary for emotional expression and release. The exercises help alleviate emotional tension by promoting relaxation and deep breathing, which are essential for emotional well-being.

4. Stress Reduction: The mind-body connection fostered by Chair Pilates serves as an excellent stress management tool. This practice enables you to release physical and emotional stress, ultimately improving your overall mental wellness.

5. Body Awareness: Chair Pilates sharpens body awareness, allowing you to better understand your physical and emotional needs. This insight supports wellness by helping you make informed choices and address concerns as they arise.

Benefits of Chair Pilates for Wellness

Chair Pilates yields a plethora of benefits that contribute to overall wellness:

1. Enhanced Posture: Chair Pilates helps improve posture by strengthening the core, spinal muscles, and upper back, reducing the risk of musculoskeletal issues related to poor posture.

2. Increased Strength and Flexibility: The practice targets muscles throughout the body, promoting strength and flexibility, which are essential for everyday functionality and well-being.

3. Improved Balance: Chair Pilates exercises challenge and enhance balance and stability, reducing the risk of falls and injuries.

4. Mindfulness and Stress Reduction: The focus on breath and concentration fosters mindfulness, aiding in stress reduction and emotional well-being.

5. Support for Rehabilitation: Chair Pilates is a gentle and supportive option for individuals recovering from injuries or surgery. It aids in rehabilitation by enhancing mobility and strength.

6. A Sense of Accomplishment: Consistent Chair Pilates practice provides a sense of accomplishment and empowerment, boosting self-esteem and overall mental well-being.

7. Holistic Wellness: Chair Pilates promotes a holistic approach to wellness, encompassing physical, mental, and emotional well-being.

The Path to Wellness with Chair Pilates

As the pursuit of wellness takes center stage in today's fast-paced world, Chair Pilates emerges as a powerful ally. Its adaptable nature makes it suitable for individuals of all ages and fitness levels, offering a gentle, yet effective approach to holistic well-being.

Chair Pilates encourages you to embark on a journey of self-discovery, where physical, mental, and emotional wellness intersect. By integrating Chair Pilates into your life, you open the door to a more balanced and vital state of being.

This journey not only encompasses the pursuit of health and fitness but also the cultivation of mindfulness and emotional harmony. Chair Pilates invites you to explore the boundless possibilities of wellness, and in doing so, to uncover a healthier, happier, and more balanced you.

Chair Pilates and Stress Reduction

In the whirlwind of our modern lives, stress has become an unwelcome companion for many. The demands of work, daily responsibilities, and the constant stream of information can leave us feeling overwhelmed and tense.

Addressing stress is not only a matter of mental well-being but is intrinsically linked to our physical health. Chair Pilates, an adaptation of the traditional Pilates method, offers a unique and effective path to reduce stress while promoting overall wellness.

This exploration delves into the profound connection between Chair Pilates and stress reduction, highlighting how this gentle yet powerful practice can bring calm to your life.

The Roots of Stress

Stress, in its many forms, can manifest as physical tension, mental fatigue, and emotional unease. Prolonged exposure to stress can lead to a range of health issues, including high blood pressure, weakened immune function, anxiety, and depression. The fast-paced nature of contemporary living often perpetuates the cycle of stress, making it essential to adopt strategies for its management and reduction.

Chair Pilates as a Stress Reduction Tool

Chair Pilates is uniquely suited to address stress due to its multifaceted approach to well-being. This practice blends physical exercise with mindfulness, fostering a holistic solution for stress reduction. Here are key elements that make Chair Pilates an effective stress reduction tool:

1. Mind-Body Connection: Chair Pilates emphasizes the connection between mind and body, focusing on mindful movements, breath control, and mental concentration. By cultivating this connection, it enables individuals to become more aware of their physical and emotional responses to stress.

2. Mindfulness and Stress Reduction: The mindfulness aspect of Chair Pilates encourages you to stay present and attentive during each exercise. This mindfulness, combined with slow and controlled movements, acts as a stress-reduction technique, effectively reducing the incessant mental chatter that often accompanies stress.

3. Physical Release: Stress often manifests as physical tension in various muscle groups, especially in the neck, shoulders, and back. Chair Pilates exercises target these areas, helping to release tension and promote relaxation.

4. Breath Control: Controlled breathing is an integral part of Chair Pilates, helping individuals establish a sense of calm and emotional balance. Deep, diaphragmatic breathing can reduce the physical symptoms of stress, such as rapid heart rate and shallow breath.

5. Posture Improvement: Many Chair Pilates exercises aim to improve posture. Enhanced posture can counteract the physical manifestations of stress, as it encourages open, upright body language, which can influence feelings of confidence and well-being.

6. Positive Self-Image: Consistent Chair Pilates practice fosters a sense of accomplishment and self-worth. This can counteract the negative self-talk that often accompanies stress, helping individuals regain a positive self-image.

7. Time for Self-Care: Engaging in Chair Pilates creates a designated time for self-care, encouraging individuals to prioritize their physical and emotional health. This practice can help individuals step away from the hustle and bustle of life and find a moment of tranquility.

The Path to Stress Reduction

Incorporating Chair Pilates into your routine can serve as a dedicated path to stress reduction. As you continue your Chair Pilates practice, you'll notice the cumulative effects of reduced tension, improved posture, and enhanced mindfulness.

These elements work in harmony to alleviate stress and promote a state of well-being. Consistency is key, and integrating Chair Pilates into your daily or weekly schedule can yield lasting stress reduction benefits.

Stress is an unavoidable facet of life, but how you choose to address and mitigate it is within your control. Chair Pilates offers a gentle, yet potent, approach to stress reduction, inviting you to embrace mindfulness, physical well-being, and self-care. By making Chair Pilates an integral part of your holistic wellness journey, you can gradually unlock a more serene and balanced way of life.

Chair Pilates for Back Pain Relief

Back pain is a pervasive and often debilitating condition that can affect people of all ages. It can be caused by various factors, including poor posture, muscle imbalances, and sedentary lifestyles.

When seeking relief from back pain, many individuals turn to Chair Pilates as a holistic and effective approach. This exploration delves into the profound connection between Chair Pilates and back pain relief, highlighting how this adaptable and gentle practice can alleviate discomfort while promoting overall spinal health.

Understanding Back Pain

Back pain can range from mild discomfort to severe, chronic pain, impacting the quality of daily life. It often occurs in the lower back but can also affect the mid and upper back. Common causes of back pain include:

- Poor posture
- Muscle imbalances
- Sedentary lifestyle
- Herniated discs
- Strained muscles
- Arthritis
- Stress and tension

The multifaceted nature of back pain necessitates a comprehensive and tailored approach to relief and rehabilitation.

Chair Pilates as a Therapeutic Tool

Chair Pilates, an adaptation of the traditional Pilates method, is celebrated for its gentle yet effective approach to improving core strength, flexibility, posture, and overall spinal health.

The chair serves as a versatile apparatus that provides support while engaging the body in a variety of exercises. This support is especially valuable for individuals seeking back pain relief, as it minimizes the strain on the spine and allows for controlled, pain-free movements. Here are key elements that make Chair Pilates a valuable tool for back pain relief:

1. **Core Strengthening:** A strong core is essential for supporting the spine and maintaining proper posture. Chair Pilates focuses on strengthening the core muscles, including the abdominals and the muscles of the lower back.

2. **Improved Posture:** Poor posture is a significant contributor to back pain. Chair Pilates incorporates exercises

that enhance spinal alignment and posture, reducing strain on the back.

3. Low-Impact Exercises: The controlled, low-impact nature of Chair Pilates minimizes the risk of exacerbating back pain. It allows individuals to engage in safe movements that gradually build strength and flexibility.

4. Muscle Balancing: Chair Pilates addresses muscle imbalances, which can lead to back pain. By targeting both the agonist and antagonist muscles, it helps create a harmonious relationship between muscle groups.

5. Range of Motion: Chair Pilates exercises promote flexibility and a healthy range of motion in the spine, which is essential for back pain relief.

6. Mind-Body Connection: Mindfulness is an integral part of Chair Pilates.

By focusing on breath and mindful movements, individuals develop a heightened awareness of their bodies, which can help alleviate back pain associated with stress and tension.

The Path to Back Pain Relief

Incorporating Chair Pilates into your routine can serve as a dedicated path to back pain relief. A structured, consistent practice allows you to gradually build strength, flexibility, and awareness while minimizing discomfort. Here's how Chair Pilates can help address back pain:

1. Pain Reduction: Chair Pilates exercises can effectively reduce pain by strengthening the core, alleviating muscle imbalances, and improving spinal alignment.

2. Prevention of Recurrence: Chair Pilates provides tools for preventing future back pain by promoting proper posture, muscle balance, and a strong core.

3. Enhanced Well-Being: As back pain diminishes, overall well-being is enhanced, as individuals experience reduced discomfort and greater freedom of movement.

4. Quality of Life: The relief from back pain allows individuals to engage in activities they may have had to forgo due to discomfort, leading to an improved quality of life.

Back pain is a common and challenging condition, but it need not control your life.

Chair Pilates offers a supportive and holistic approach to back pain relief, helping you regain control over your physical health and well-being.

By integrating Chair Pilates into your routine, you embark on a journey toward greater comfort, flexibility, and spinal health.

This journey holds the promise of a life with reduced back pain and increased mobility.

Chair Pilates for Improved Posture

Posture is more than a matter of aesthetics; it is a reflection of your overall well-being. A hunched or misaligned posture can lead to a myriad of physical issues and discomfort. Fortunately, Chair Pilates offers a dynamic and accessible approach to enhancing your posture.

In this exploration, we delve into the profound connection between Chair Pilates and improved posture, emphasizing how this adaptable and gentle practice can help you stand tall and feel your best.

Understanding the Importance of Posture

Good posture is a fundamental component of physical well-being. It involves the proper alignment of the spine, which supports the body's structures and ensures their efficient functioning. When posture is compromised, it can result in various issues, including:

- Muscular imbalances
- Increased risk of injury
- Back and neck pain
- Reduced lung capacity
- Reduced circulation
- Digestive issues
- Reduced self-confidence

Recognizing the far-reaching implications of posture on overall health underscores the significance of addressing postural concerns.

Chair Pilates as a Posture-Enhancing Practice

Chair Pilates, an adaptation of traditional Pilates, offers a distinctive approach to posture improvement. The chair serves as a versatile and supportive apparatus that facilitates controlled movements and precise alignment.

This makes Chair Pilates a suitable choice for individuals seeking to enhance their posture gently and effectively. Here are key elements that make Chair Pilates a valuable tool for posture improvement:

1. Core Strengthening: A strong core is integral to maintaining an upright posture. Chair Pilates focuses on strengthening the core muscles, including the abdominals and the muscles of the lower back.

2. Spinal Alignment: Chair Pilates incorporates exercises that promote proper spinal alignment. These movements help the spine find its natural curve and prevent the development of poor posture.

3. Low-Impact Exercises: Chair Pilates is a low-impact practice that minimizes the risk of injury. This allows individuals to engage in safe movements that gradually enhance postural integrity.

4. Muscle Balancing: Chair Pilates addresses muscle imbalances, which can contribute to poor posture. By targeting both the agonist and antagonist muscles, it helps create symmetry in muscle development.

5. Mind-Body Connection: Mindfulness is a fundamental part of Chair Pilates. By concentrating on breath and mindful movements, individuals develop an enhanced awareness of their bodies, which can lead to more conscious and aligned posture.

The Journey to Improved Posture

Incorporating Chair Pilates into your routine can serve as a dedicated path to improved posture. With consistent practice, you can gradually build strength, flexibility, and awareness while transforming your posture. Here's how Chair Pilates can help enhance your posture:

1. Alignment: Chair Pilates exercises focus on spinal alignment, helping you rediscover your natural posture and counteracting the effects of poor habits.

2. Strength: A stronger core and supportive muscles are essential for maintaining an upright posture. Chair Pilates builds this strength gradually and effectively.

3. Mindful Posture: Chair Pilates fosters mindfulness, enabling you to carry the principles of proper posture into your daily life.

4. Muscle Symmetry: Addressing muscle imbalances through Chair Pilates promotes symmetry and balanced development, which is crucial for posture improvement.

5. Pain Reduction: As posture improves, individuals often experience reduced discomfort, particularly in the neck, shoulders, and lower back.

The Rewards of Improved Posture

Enhancing your posture is more than a cosmetic change; it is an investment in your overall well-being. The rewards of improved posture include:

- Enhanced physical comfort
- Reduced risk of musculoskeletal issues
- Greater self-confidence
- Improved lung capacity and circulation
- Better digestive function
- A sense of vitality and well-being

Chair Pilates serves as a transformative and accessible tool for those seeking improved posture and the associated benefits. By incorporating Chair Pilates into your routine, you embark on a journey toward enhanced alignment, strength, and mindfulness.

This journey promises not only a more upright and balanced posture but also a healthier and more vital you.

Chair Pilates for Increased Flexibility

Flexibility is an essential component of physical well-being, enhancing your range of motion and reducing the risk of injury. Chair Pilates, an adaptive form of the traditional Pilates method, offers a unique and gentle approach to improving flexibility.

This exploration uncovers the profound connection between Chair Pilates and increased flexibility, highlighting how this versatile and accessible practice can help you achieve a more supple and mobile body.

The Significance of Flexibility

Flexibility, often associated with graceful dancers and yogis, is a crucial aspect of physical wellness that extends far beyond aesthetics. Adequate flexibility supports overall health and well-being by:

- Enhancing range of motion: Improved flexibility allows you to move your joints and muscles through

their full range of motion, promoting better posture
and reducing the risk of injury.

- Alleviating muscular tension: Flexible muscles are
  less prone to tension and discomfort. A supple body
  can reduce the occurrence of aches and pains.

- Encouraging relaxation: The gentle stretching
  involved in flexibility exercises can promote
  relaxation and relieve stress.

- Promoting circulation: Flexible muscles and joints
  facilitate better circulation, ensuring your body
  receives the nutrients it needs.

Chair Pilates as a Flexibility-Enhancing Practice

Chair Pilates introduces an adaptable and effective approach
to increasing flexibility. The chair serves as a supportive
apparatus that allows for controlled and precise movements.

This supportive element is particularly valuable for
individuals who may require assistance due to physical
limitations or those who prefer a gentle introduction to
flexibility training. Key elements make Chair Pilates a
valuable tool for enhancing flexibility:

1. Low-Impact Movements: Chair Pilates is a low-impact practice that minimizes the risk of injury, making it suitable for individuals of all fitness levels and ages.

2. Controlled Stretching: The controlled and precise nature of Chair Pilates stretches targets muscles and joints safely, gradually promoting increased flexibility.

3. Mind-Body Connection: Mindfulness is an integral part of Chair Pilates. Concentrating on breath and mindful movements encourages awareness and a deeper connection between the body and the mind.

4. Spinal Flexibility: Chair Pilates exercises often involve spinal stretches that enhance flexibility along the length of the spine, contributing to better posture and overall suppleness.

The Journey to Increased Flexibility

Incorporating Chair Pilates into your routine can serve as a dedicated path to increased flexibility. Through consistent practice, you can gradually enhance your flexibility, leading to a more supple and mobile body. Here's how Chair Pilates can help you on your journey to greater flexibility:

1. Muscle Lengthening: Chair Pilates exercises focus on elongating muscles, aiding in improved flexibility.

2. Range of Motion: Controlled movements help you gradually increase your range of motion, allowing for greater flexibility in joints and muscles.

3. Mindful Stretching: The mindfulness aspect of Chair Pilates encourages you to stay present during stretching exercises, helping you become more aware of your body's limits and progress.

4. Reduced Muscle Tension: Chair Pilates can alleviate muscular tension, which is often a barrier to achieving greater flexibility.

The Rewards of Increased Flexibility

The journey to increased flexibility offers numerous rewards, including:

- Greater range of motion and mobility
- Reduced muscular tension and discomfort
- Enhanced posture and body awareness
- Reduced risk of injury

- Enhanced relaxation and stress reduction
- An overall sense of well-being

Chair Pilates serves as a transformative and adaptable tool for those seeking increased flexibility and the associated benefits.

By incorporating Chair Pilates into your routine, you embark on a journey toward a more supple, mobile, and balanced body. This journey promises not only an increased range of motion but also a healthier and more vital you.

Chair Pilates for Overall Well-being

In our quest for overall well-being, it's essential to embrace a holistic approach that addresses the body, mind, and spirit. Chair Pilates, an accessible and adaptable form of the traditional Pilates method, offers a comprehensive path to achieve and maintain a sense of vitality and equilibrium.

This exploration dives into the profound connection between Chair Pilates and overall well-being, highlighting how this gentle yet dynamic practice can enhance your physical health, mental clarity, and emotional balance.

Defining Overall Well-being

Overall well-being encompasses more than just physical health; it encompasses a state of complete harmony that includes mental, emotional, and social well-being. This holistic approach acknowledges the interconnectedness of these dimensions, emphasizing their collective influence on one's quality of life. Key elements of overall well-being include:

1. Physical Health: Robust physical health involves proper nutrition, regular exercise, and maintenance of bodily systems.

2. Mental Clarity: A sharp mind that's free from undue stress and mental fog is essential for overall well-being.

3. Emotional Balance: Emotional health is crucial, as it influences one's relationships and outlook on life.

4. Social Connection: Healthy relationships and a supportive social network are integral to overall well-being.

Chair Pilates as a Holistic Practice

Chair Pilates offers a unique and inclusive approach to overall well-being.

This practice aligns with the fundamental principles of Pilates, emphasizing concentration, control, centering, precision, and breath.

By embracing these principles, Chair Pilates nurtures the connection between the body and the mind, promoting mindfulness and emotional balance.

Key elements that make Chair Pilates a valuable tool for overall well-being include:

1. Physical Fitness: Chair Pilates provides a comprehensive approach to physical fitness, focusing on core strength, flexibility, balance, and posture. These elements are vital for sustaining physical well-being and preventing musculoskeletal issues.

2. Mindfulness: Chair Pilates encourages you to stay present during each movement, fostering mindfulness that can be applied to daily life, reducing stress, and enhancing mental clarity.

3. Emotional Release: The controlled and gentle movements in Chair Pilates create an opportunity to release emotional tension, promote relaxation, and manage stress.

4. Improved Posture: Chair Pilates exercises often emphasize posture improvement, helping you stand tall and maintain alignment, reducing the risk of musculoskeletal issues.

5. Muscle Balance: Chair Pilates addresses muscle imbalances, creating a harmonious relationship between muscle groups, which is essential for overall well-being.

The Path to Overall Well-being

Incorporating Chair Pilates into your routine can serve as a dedicated path to overall well-being. With consistent practice, you can gradually build physical strength, flexibility, mental clarity, and emotional balance.

Here's how Chair Pilates can help enhance your overall well-being:

1. Physical Vitality: Chair Pilates improves physical fitness, contributing to overall health and vitality.

2. Mindful Living: The mindfulness cultivated in Chair Pilates extends beyond the mat, helping you approach life with greater awareness and clarity.

3. Stress Reduction: Chair Pilates offers a gentle and effective means of stress reduction, promoting emotional balance and reducing the risk of stress-related health issues.

4. Healthy Posture: Improved posture through Chair Pilates enhances physical comfort and supports overall well-being.

5. Positive Outlook: Chair Pilates fosters a sense of accomplishment and self-worth, contributing to a positive outlook on life.

6. Social Connection: The Chair Pilates community provides social connections, supporting overall well-being.

Chair Pilates offers a holistic and adaptable tool for those seeking overall well-being, bridging the gap between physical, mental, and emotional health.

By incorporating Chair Pilates into your routine, you embark on a transformative journey that promises a life characterized by vitality, mindfulness, and emotional balance.

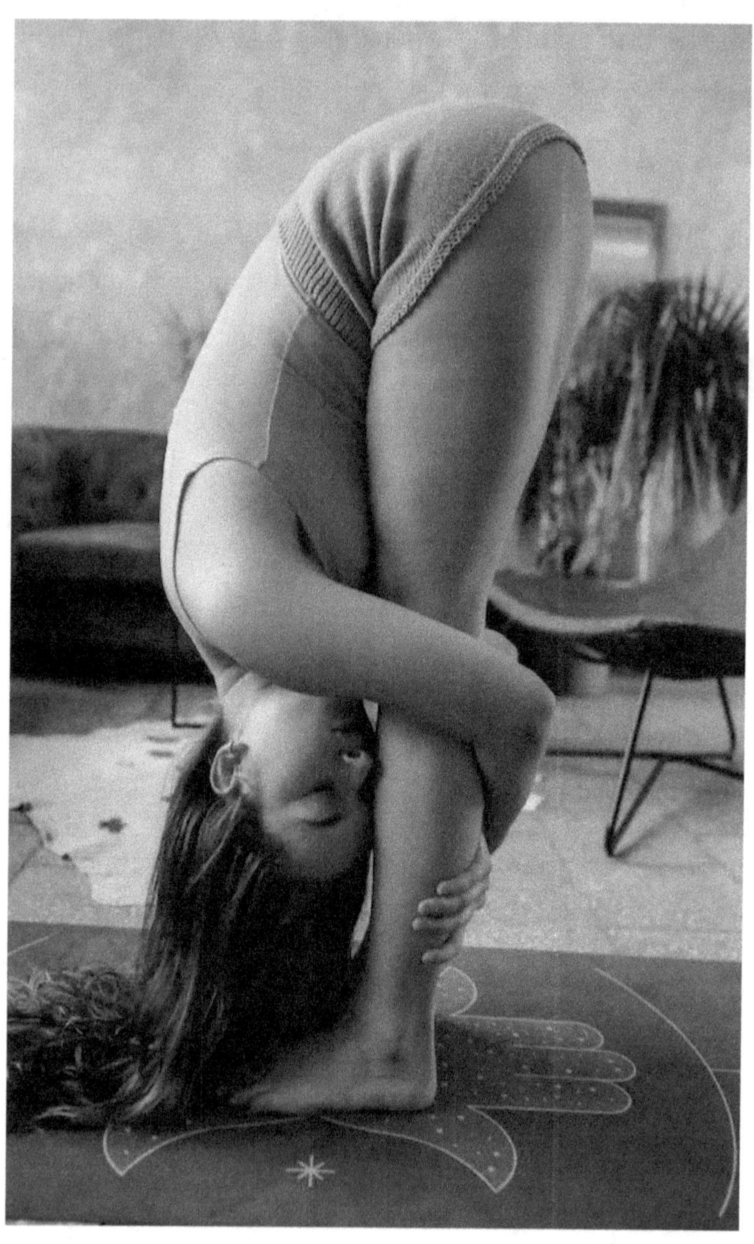

CHAPTER FIVE

Chair Pilates Progression and Advanced Techniques

Chair Pilates is a versatile and adaptable form of the traditional Pilates method that offers a broad spectrum of benefits to individuals of all fitness levels.

While Chair Pilates is accessible to beginners, it is equally conducive to progression and advanced techniques. In this comprehensive introduction, we delve into the world of Chair Pilates progression, exploring how practitioners can take their practice to the next level and explore advanced techniques to enhance their physical and mental well-being.

The Foundational Principles of Chair Pilates

Chair Pilates adheres to the foundational principles of Pilates, which include concentration, control, centering, precision, and breath. These principles create a strong mind-body connection and serve as the cornerstone of any Pilates practice. As practitioners become more comfortable with these principles, they can expand their repertoire and delve into more advanced techniques while maintaining the integrity of the practice.

The Journey of Progression

Chair Pilates progression is an evolution of the practice, representing an individual's journey from a novice to an advanced practitioner. This progression is marked by the development of core strength, flexibility, posture, and mindfulness. As individuals grow in their practice, they become more adept at maintaining proper form, integrating advanced exercises, and exploring nuanced techniques. The progression of Chair Pilates often follows a pattern:

1. Foundation: Beginners start with foundational exercises that introduce the core principles of Chair Pilates. These exercises focus on building a strong core, improving posture, and developing awareness.

2. Intermediate: As practitioners gain confidence and strength, they move on to intermediate exercises that involve more complex movements and greater demands on the muscles.

3. Advanced: Advanced Chair Pilates techniques challenge practitioners with intricate exercises that require a high degree of control, strength, and flexibility.

These exercises often push the boundaries of what individuals thought possible in their practice.

Advanced Techniques in Chair Pilates

Advanced Chair Pilates techniques expand upon the foundational and intermediate exercises, offering a diverse range of challenging movements. These advanced techniques require precise control, heightened concentration, and a deep understanding of the body-mind connection. Here are some examples of advanced Chair Pilates techniques:

1. Inversions: Advanced Chair Pilates exercises can involve partial or full inversions, where practitioners lift their legs above their heads while maintaining balance and control.

2. Isometric Holds: Isometric exercises focus on holding a position without movement. Advanced Chair Pilates incorporates isometric holds that challenge core strength and endurance.

3. Dynamic Balancing: Advanced practitioners may explore dynamic balancing exercises that involve intricate movements while balancing on the chair.

4. Resistance Bands: Incorporating resistance bands into Chair Pilates can add an extra layer of challenge, enhancing strength and flexibility.

5. Spinal Articulation: Advanced Chair Pilates often includes complex exercises that articulate and mobilize the spine in multiple directions, promoting spinal health and flexibility.

The Benefits of Chair Pilates Progression and Advanced Techniques

The progression and integration of advanced techniques in Chair Pilates offer a host of benefits, including:

- Enhanced Core Strength: Advanced techniques challenge the core muscles more intensely, leading to greater core strength and stability.
- Improved Flexibility: Advanced movements promote increased flexibility and range of motion.
- Mental Engagement: As practitioners advance, Chair Pilates requires heightened mental engagement, fostering greater mindfulness and concentration.
- Elevated Postural Awareness: Advanced techniques contribute to improved posture and alignment.

- Physical Challenge: The increased intensity of advanced exercises offers a satisfying physical challenge, pushing practitioners to their limits and helping them discover their true potential.
- Holistic Well-being: Chair Pilates progression and advanced techniques support holistic well-being by enhancing physical health, mental clarity, and emotional balance.

Chair Pilates progression and the exploration of advanced techniques represent a dynamic and transformative journey. Practitioners who commit to this path discover the depth and breadth of Chair Pilates, unlocking the potential for physical, mental, and emotional well-being.

As individuals evolve in their practice, they tap into the profound benefits that Chair Pilates offers, enhancing their quality of life and realizing their full potential in this versatile and adaptable discipline.

Building Strength and Flexibility

Chair Pilates is an excellent method for building both strength and flexibility in a gentle and controlled manner.

Whether you're a beginner looking to lay the foundation or an advanced practitioner seeking to enhance your physical capabilities, Chair Pilates offers a diverse range of exercises and techniques to help you achieve your goals.

In this exploration, we'll delve into the ways in which Chair Pilates can be harnessed to build strength and flexibility, offering a comprehensive understanding of its potential benefits.

The Marriage of Strength and Flexibility

Strength and flexibility are often seen as contrasting aspects of physical fitness, but in reality, they complement each other. To achieve a balanced and healthy body, it's essential to cultivate both. Here's how they intertwine:

- Strength: A strong body provides support and stability for your daily activities, protecting you from injury and enhancing your overall physical performance.

- Flexibility: A flexible body allows for a broader range of motion in joints and muscles, which is essential for activities that require agility and fluidity.

Chair Pilates is an ideal approach for developing this dynamic balance because it incorporates both elements into its exercises.

Building Strength with Chair Pilates

Chair Pilates is a versatile method for building strength. It focuses on developing the core muscles, including the abdominals and lower back, which are essential for supporting the spine and maintaining proper posture. Here's how Chair Pilates helps build strength:

1. Core Engagement: Many Chair Pilates exercises involve core engagement, strengthening the deep abdominal muscles and improving stability.

2. Resistance: Some Chair Pilates exercises incorporate resistance bands or additional props, adding an extra layer of challenge to build muscular strength.

3. Balancing Acts: Balancing exercises, such as those performed on the chair, strengthen not only the core but also the stabilizing muscles throughout the body.

4. Bodyweight Exercises: Chair Pilates utilizes bodyweight resistance effectively, allowing you to build strength without the need for external weights.

Building Flexibility with Chair Pilates

Flexibility is a vital component of Chair Pilates, and it's woven into the very fabric of the practice. Chair Pilates enhances flexibility by:

1. Controlled Stretching: Chair Pilates incorporates controlled stretching exercises that help lengthen muscles and improve flexibility.

2. Spinal Mobilization: Many Chair Pilates exercises focus on spinal articulation and mobilization, promoting flexibility along the length of the spine.

3. Range of Motion: Controlled, precise movements in Chair Pilates gradually increase your range of motion, leading to greater flexibility in both joints and muscles.

4. Mindful Stretching: The mindfulness aspect of Chair Pilates encourages you to stay present during stretching exercises, helping you become more aware of your body's limits and progress.

The Benefits of Strength and Flexibility in Chair Pilates

The interplay between strength and flexibility in Chair Pilates offers a host of benefits:

- Enhanced Posture: Improved strength and flexibility contribute to better posture, reducing the risk of musculoskeletal issues related to poor alignment.

- Injury Prevention: Strong and flexible muscles are less prone to injury, making Chair Pilates an excellent practice for injury prevention.

- Increased Range of Motion: The dynamic range of motion achieved in Chair Pilates enhances physical capabilities for daily activities and sports.

- Mind-Body Connection: Building both strength and flexibility deepens the mind-body connection, fostering greater awareness and control.

- Reduced Muscle Tension: Flexible muscles are less likely to become tense and tight, leading to reduced discomfort and pain.

- Balance and Agility: Strength and flexibility combine to enhance balance, agility, and overall physical performance.

Chair Pilates offers a dynamic platform for building strength and flexibility in a controlled and mindful manner. Whether you're just beginning or looking to advance your practice, the adaptability of Chair Pilates provides a nurturing environment to cultivate these essential physical attributes.

By incorporating Chair Pilates into your routine, you embark on a transformative journey that promises a healthier, more balanced, and agile you.

Advanced Chair Pilates Exercises

Chair Pilates, an adaptable and holistic form of exercise, offers a broad spectrum of exercises suitable for individuals of all fitness levels.

As you advance in your practice, you'll find a wealth of advanced Chair Pilates exercises that challenge your strength, flexibility, and control. These exercises, designed for those seeking a more profound Pilates experience, enable you to elevate your practice and explore the full potential of your body and mind.

In this exploration, we'll delve into some advanced Chair Pilates exercises that are designed to challenge and inspire.

1. The Teaser on the Chair: The Teaser on the Chair is an advanced exercise that enhances core strength, balance, and control. To perform this exercise:

- Sit on the edge of the chair with your knees bent and feet flat on the floor.
- Place your hands on the sides of the chair seat.
- Lift your feet off the floor, extending your legs forward and keeping them parallel to the ground.
- Inhale as you extend your arms forward, reaching them toward your feet.
- Exhale as you round your spine, rolling back slowly until your back is parallel to the ground.
- Inhale to maintain the position.
- Exhale to roll back up to the starting position.
- Repeat for a set number of repetitions.

2. The Mermaid Stretch:

The Mermaid Stretch on the Chair is a beautiful exercise that promotes flexibility, spinal articulation, and balance. To perform this exercise:

- Sit on the chair facing to the right with your knees bent and your feet off the ground.

- Place your right hand on the seat and your left hand on the top of the backrest.
- Inhale to lengthen your spine, then exhale to side-bend to the right, lifting your hips off the seat.
- Inhale to hold the side-bend position.
- Exhale to return to the starting position.
- Perform the exercise on both sides for a balanced workout.

3. The Swan Dive on the Chair: The Swan Dive on the Chair is an advanced exercise that enhances upper body and core strength while promoting spinal extension. To perform this exercise:

- Sit on the chair facing forward with your hands on the front edge of the seat.
- Inhale to lift your chest, extending your spine and leaning slightly back.
- Exhale as you lift your feet off the ground, extending your legs and arms forward.
- Inhale to hold the position.
- Exhale to return to the starting position.

4. The High Chair Knee Stretch Series: The High Chair Knee Stretch Series is a series of advanced exercises that challenge core strength and balance. To perform these exercises:

- Sit on the chair facing forward with your knees bent, feet off the ground, and your hands on the front edge of the seat.
- Lift your feet off the ground, extending your legs forward.
- Inhale as you extend your legs, and then exhale to bring your knees to your chest, rounding your spine.
- Repeat this movement for a set number of repetitions.
- You can also add variations, such as lifting one leg at a time or performing a bicycle motion.

5. The Horseback on the Chair: The Horseback on the Chair is an advanced exercise that enhances core strength and balance. To perform this exercise:

- Sit on the chair facing forward with your knees bent and your feet off the ground.
- Place your hands on the front edge of the seat.

- Inhale to lift your chest and extend your spine.
- Exhale as you lift your feet off the ground and extend your legs, creating a straight line from your head to your heels.
- Inhale to maintain the position.
- Exhale to return to the starting position.

These advanced Chair Pilates exercises are designed to challenge your physical and mental capacities while deepening your practice. As you progress, it's crucial to maintain proper form and control to avoid injury.

It's recommended to work with a qualified Pilates instructor who can guide you through these advanced exercises and tailor them to your specific needs and goals. Advanced Chair Pilates exercises offer a pathway to further enhance your physical abilities, mindfulness, and overall well-being.

Chair Pilates for Specific Goals

Chair Pilates is a versatile and adaptive form of exercise that can be tailored to help you achieve specific fitness and well-being goals. Whether you're aiming to improve core strength, increase flexibility, enhance posture, or manage stress, Chair Pilates offers a variety of exercises and techniques to target your specific objectives.

In this exploration, we'll delve into how Chair Pilates can be customized to address distinct goals and support your journey to better health and vitality.

1. Core Strengthening with Chair Pilates:

Core strength is a cornerstone of physical well-being, providing support for your spine and helping you maintain proper posture. Chair Pilates offers a range of exercises to strengthen your core:

- Hundred on the Chair: This exercise involves pumping your arms while holding a "V" position with your legs, engaging the core throughout.
- Knee Stretch Series: This series focuses on bringing your knees toward your chest from a plank position, targeting the abdominal muscles.
- Twisting Exercises: Twisting movements on the chair work the obliques, enhancing core stability.

By incorporating these exercises into your Chair Pilates routine, you can develop a strong and resilient core.

2. Increasing Flexibility with Chair Pilates

Flexibility is vital for maintaining a broad range of motion and preventing injuries. Chair Pilates offers numerous stretching exercises to increase flexibility:

- Spinal Articulation: This exercise focuses on mobilizing the spine in multiple directions, promoting spinal flexibility.
- Teaser on the Chair: The Teaser exercise challenges the flexibility of the back and hamstrings while engaging the core.
- Mermaid Stretch: This exercise enhances lateral spinal flexibility and opens up the sides of the body.

Regularly incorporating these stretching exercises into your Chair Pilates practice can lead to improved flexibility.

3. Posture Improvement through Chair Pilates: Good posture is essential for overall well-being, reducing the risk of musculoskeletal issues and promoting a confident and poised appearance. Chair Pilates exercises for better posture include:

- Saw Exercise: The Saw exercise encourages spinal rotation and stretches the back of the legs, helping to improve posture.

- Swan Dive on the Chair: This exercise focuses on spinal extension, which is essential for countering poor posture.

- The Mermaid Stretch: The Mermaid Stretch promotes lateral flexibility and strengthens the core, both of which contribute to better alignment.

By regularly practicing these exercises, you can enhance your posture and reduce the risk of discomfort associated with poor alignment.

4. Stress Management with Chair Pilates: Chair Pilates incorporates mindfulness and controlled breathing, making it a valuable tool for stress reduction. Specific Chair Pilates exercises for managing stress include:

- Breathing Techniques: Chair Pilates incorporates various breathing exercises to enhance relaxation and mental clarity.

- Mindfulness and Concentration: The mindful movements and concentration required in Chair

Pilates encourage mental focus, reducing stress and promoting emotional balance.

By integrating Chair Pilates into your routine, you can reduce stress and find greater peace of mind.

5. Upper Body and Lower Body Workouts: Chair Pilates can be customized to provide targeted workouts for the upper body and lower body:

- Upper Body Exercises: To strengthen the upper body, you can incorporate exercises like push-ups, tricep dips, and arm circles using the chair as support.
- Lower Body Exercises: For lower body strengthening, you can perform exercises like leg lifts, squats, and leg extensions using the chair.

Tailoring your Chair Pilates routine to focus on the upper or lower body allows you to meet specific fitness goals.

Customizing Chair Pilates to your specific goals is a flexible and effective approach to improving your physical and mental well-being.

To make the most of your customized Chair Pilates routine, consider working with a qualified Pilates instructor who can provide guidance and adjustments tailored to your objectives. Chair Pilates offers a pathway to better health and vitality by addressing your unique goals and helping you achieve a greater sense of well-being.

Maintaining a Regular Practice

Maintaining a regular Chair Pilates practice is essential for reaping the full benefits of this versatile and adaptive exercise method. Consistency is key to achieving your fitness and well-being goals, whether they involve core strength, flexibility, posture improvement, stress management, or other specific objectives. In this exploration, we'll delve into strategies and tips to help you maintain a consistent Chair Pilates practice and integrate it seamlessly into your daily routine.

1. Establish a Routine:

One of the most effective ways to maintain a regular Chair Pilates practice is to establish a routine. Choose a specific time each day or week when you can dedicate yourself to your practice. Consistency makes it easier to form a habit, and your body and mind will come to expect and anticipate your Pilates sessions.

2. Set Realistic Goals: Setting achievable and realistic goals can help you stay motivated and committed to your Chair Pilates practice. Whether you want to improve core strength, increase flexibility, or manage stress, having clear and attainable goals gives you a sense of purpose and direction.

3. Find Accountability: Accountability can be a powerful motivator. Consider practicing Chair Pilates with a friend or joining a Pilates class where you're held accountable by an instructor and fellow participants. You can also set up regular check-ins or progress reports to keep yourself on track.

4. Create a Dedicated Space: Designate a specific space for your Chair Pilates practice. Having a dedicated area where your chair and exercise equipment are readily available makes it more convenient to engage in your practice regularly. This space can serve as a visual reminder of your commitment.

5. Stay Mindful and Present: Mindfulness is a fundamental aspect of Chair Pilates, and it's essential to carry this mindfulness into your daily life. Stay present and aware of your body, posture, and alignment as you go about your day.

This mindfulness will naturally extend to your practice and help you stay engaged and consistent.

6. Mix Up Your Routine: Variety keeps your Chair Pilates practice fresh and exciting. Experiment with different exercises, explore advanced techniques, and add new elements to your routine. This variety can prevent boredom and keep you motivated.

7. Track Your Progress: Document your Chair Pilates journey by keeping a journal or using a fitness app. Record your goals, the exercises you've performed, and any changes you've noticed in your body and well-being. Tracking your progress can be motivating and rewarding.

8. Listen to Your Body: Listening to your body is crucial for maintaining a regular Chair Pilates practice. If you're feeling fatigued or experiencing discomfort, it's okay to take a break or modify your routine. Pay attention to your body's signals and adjust your practice as needed to avoid overexertion or injury.

9. Stay Committed to Self-Care: Chair Pilates is not only about physical exercise but also a form of self-care. Remind yourself of the physical and mental benefits you gain from your practice, and make self-care a priority in your life. Regularly practicing Chair Pilates is an act of self-love and well-being.

10. Seek Professional Guidance: Consider working with a qualified Chair Pilates instructor. They can provide guidance, correct your form, and offer personalized exercises that align with your specific goals. Professional guidance ensures that you're practicing Chair Pilates safely and effectively.

Maintaining a regular Chair Pilates practice is an investment in your physical and mental well-being. By implementing these strategies and tips, you can establish a consistent routine, achieve your goals, and enjoy the numerous benefits that Chair Pilates has to offer.

Continuing Your Chair Pilates Journey

Continuing your Chair Pilates journey is a rewarding and transformative experience that allows you to build upon your existing skills and further enhance your physical and mental well-being. As you progress, you'll discover new challenges and opportunities for growth within this adaptable exercise method. In this exploration, we'll delve into how to continue your Chair Pilates journey, whether you're a beginner looking to advance your practice or an experienced practitioner seeking to deepen your understanding and capabilities.

1. Advanced Techniques and Exercises: As you become more experienced in Chair Pilates, consider exploring advanced techniques and exercises. These movements challenge your strength, flexibility, and control, taking your practice to a new level. Some advanced exercises include the Teaser on the Chair, Swan Dive on the Chair, and the Horseback on the Chair.

2. Personalized Practice: Tailor your Chair Pilates routine to your specific needs and objectives. Whether you're looking to target core strength, increase flexibility, or enhance your posture, personalize your practice by selecting exercises that align with your goals. A qualified Pilates instructor can help you create a personalized routine.

3. Pilates Variations: Explore different variations of Chair Pilates, such as Mat Pilates and Reformer Pilates. Integrating these variations into your practice can provide a well-rounded Pilates experience and introduce new elements to challenge your body and mind.

4. Consistency and Routine: Maintain a consistent practice routine. Regularity is essential for maximizing the benefits of Chair Pilates. Set aside dedicated time for your practice and stick to it as closely as possible.

5. Ongoing Learning: Stay open to continuous learning and improvement. Attend workshops, seminars, or classes led by experienced Pilates instructors to expand your knowledge and refine your techniques. There's always more to discover and refine within the practice of Chair Pilates.

6. Mindful Practice: Focus on the mindfulness aspect of Chair Pilates. Stay present during your practice, paying attention to your breath, movements, and sensations. This mindfulness deepens your mind-body connection and enhances your overall well-being.

7. Building Strength and Flexibility: Continue building strength and flexibility, as these are foundational elements of Chair Pilates. Experiment with exercises that challenge your core, stretch your muscles, and promote balance.

Building and maintaining these attributes contribute to your overall physical health.

8. Goal Setting: Set clear and achievable goals for your Chair Pilates practice. Having specific objectives provides direction and motivation. Whether you're aiming to perfect a specific exercise or achieve a certain level of flexibility, goals give your practice purpose.

9. Professional Guidance: Work with a qualified Pilates instructor who can provide expert guidance, correct your form, and help you advance your practice safely. Their expertise and feedback are invaluable as you continue your Chair Pilates journey.

10. Listen to Your Body: Above all, listen to your body. Your body is the best indicator of what is right for you. If you're feeling fatigued or experiencing discomfort, it's okay to adjust your practice or take a rest day. Honoring your body's signals is essential for a sustainable and enjoyable Pilates journey.Continuing your Chair Pilates journey is an ongoing process of growth and self-discovery. With dedication, consistency, and a commitment to your well-being, you can deepen your practice, achieve your goals, and unlock the profound benefits that Chair Pilates offers.

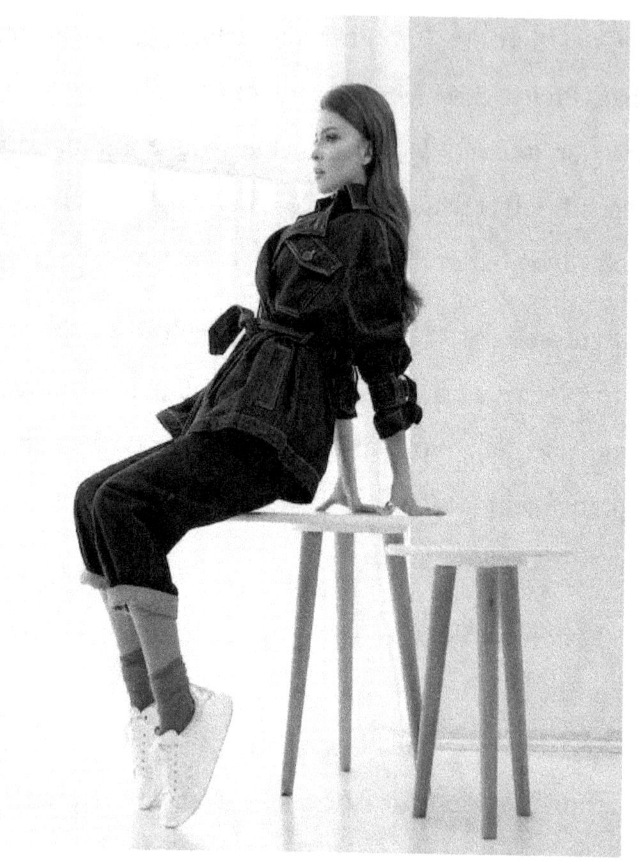

CONCLUSION

In conclusion, Chair Pilates for beginners is a remarkable fitness and well-being journey that offers numerous benefits and rewards. As we've explored, this adaptable and holistic exercise method provides a gentle yet effective path to physical strength, flexibility, posture improvement, stress management, and overall vitality.

For those taking their first steps into the world of Chair Pilates, it's a journey marked by discovery, growth, and a profound connection between the body and mind.

For beginners, Chair Pilates is an accessible and welcoming practice. Its emphasis on fundamental principles, such as concentration, control, centering, precision, and breath, ensures a solid foundation for those new to the method. These principles guide practitioners in cultivating mindfulness and deepening their mind-body connection.

Chair Pilates introduces a diverse range of exercises, catering to all fitness levels, and enabling beginners to progress at their own pace.

This adaptability makes Chair Pilates an inclusive choice for individuals of all backgrounds and abilities, ensuring that anyone can embark on this transformative journey.

The benefits of Chair Pilates for beginners are abundant. Enhanced core strength, improved flexibility, and better posture provide a solid foundation for a healthier and more balanced body. The mindfulness and controlled breathing techniques promote stress management and mental clarity, offering a path to emotional well-being.

As beginners in Chair Pilates continue their journey, they have the opportunity to explore more advanced techniques, personalize their practice, and set specific goals. With consistency, dedication, and professional guidance, they can deepen their practice and unlock the full potential of this versatile exercise method.

In essence, Chair Pilates for beginners is a holistic approach to health and wellness that supports the pursuit of physical fitness, mental clarity, and emotional balance. It is a journey of self-discovery and empowerment, inviting individuals to connect with their bodies, explore their potential, and unlock a greater sense of well-being.

www.ingramcontent.com/pod-product-compliance
Lightning Source LLC
Chambersburg PA
CBHW050825260726
48660CB00004B/1613